Contributing Authors

SO-BNZ-868

Dr. Gregory Allen
Assistant Professor
Pennsylvania State University
MHAUS Hotline Consultant
Department of Anesthesia
Hershey, Pennsylvania

Dr. Wayne Barry
Assistant Professor
University of Ottawa
Department of Anesthesia
Ottawa Hospital - Civic Campus

Dr. Greg Bryson
Assistant Professor
University of Ottawa
Department of Anesthesia
Director Preadmission Unit
Ottawa Hospital - Civic Campus

Dr. Robert Cirone
Staff Anesthesiologist
Department of Anesthesia
St. Joseph's Hospital
Toronto

Dr. Robert Elliot
Assistant Professor
University of Ottawa
Department of Anesthesia
Ottawa Hospital - General Campus

Dr. John Kitts
Associate Professor Anesthesia
University of Ottawa
Vice President Medical Affairs
Ottawa Hospital

Dr. Anne Lui
Assistant Professor
University of Ottawa
Department of Anesthesia
Ottawa Hospital - Civic Campus

Dr. John Penning
Assistant Professor
University of Ottawa
Director of the Acute Pain Service
Department of Anesthesia
Ottawa Hospital - Civic Campus

Dr. Gordon Reid
Assistant Professor
University of Ottawa
Director Malignant Hyperthermia
Investigation Unit
Department of Anesthesia
Ottawa Hospital - Civic Campus

Dr. Linda Robinson
Assistant Professor
University of Ottawa
Department of Anesthesia
Ottawa Hospital - Civic Campus

Introduction

Specialists in the fields of medicine and surgery may ask why medical students should be exposed to the specialty of anesthesia. We believe that there are basic concepts and technical skills that every physician should possess, and that these concepts and skills are best taught by our specialty.

Medical school curricula across North America are repeatedly criticized for lacking the teaching of both acute and chronic pain management. In addition, students who pursue a career in surgery, emergency medicine or internal medicine are expected to have the skills to manage a patient's airway. However, they usually have had no formal teaching in these basic skills. Finally, medical school curricula in North America are rapidly changing. Students are now asked to commit themselves to a specialty during the third year of their medical school training. We believe that this process is unfair. We also recognize that a student with no prior exposure to anesthesia is unlikely to choose anesthesia as a career.

This manual was written with contributing authors from the Departments of Anesthesia at the Ottawa Civic and General Hospitals for medical students spending two weeks of their clinical rotation in the specialty of anesthesia. Six specific objectives are used to focus the students reading. The text is highlighted by two asterisks (**) for material that is essential and that the student must know, and one asterisks (*) for material which the student should know. All other material is provided for background reading which the student may know. The manual is to be used as a primary reference for lectures on monitoring in anesthesia, and on acute and chronic pain management. The problem-based tutorial question will also be on material covered in this manual.

The student who completes the anesthesia rotation should have acquired confidence in airway management skills including mask ventilation and tracheal intubation, as well as securing intravenous access. Important concepts for the student to attain during their rotation include:

1. Preoperative assessment.
2. Basic principles of managing acute and chronic pain disorders.
3. The appropriate use of local anaesthetic agents.
4. Analgesic options for women in labour.
5. Basic neonatal assessment and resuscitation.
6. Intravenous fluid and blood component therapy including the potential complications of a blood product transfusion.

Patrick Sullivan MD, FRCPC
Assistant Professor
University of Ottawa,
Resident Program Director
Department of Anesthesia
University of Ottawa

Preface

The first public demonstration of ether was by W.T.G. Morton in the Etherdome of the Massachusetts General Hospital in 1846. Ether anaesthesia became widely available and would soon be followed by chloroform and nitrous oxide. Surgeons were not particular about who poured the ether or chloroform so long as someone was there to do the job. It was not until the early 1920's that physicians began to show interest in anaesthesia as a specialty. By the end of World War II the infant specialty was firmly established and university training programs began.

The emphasis has traditionally been on postgraduate teaching. Why has undergraduate anaesthesia teaching been neglected or de-emphasized? It was because the medical school curriculum was controlled by older, traditional disciplines that were unwilling to relinquish time for competing specialties. This was complicated by the fact that anaesthetists originally worked only in the operating room, and found it difficult to be freed from that responsibility to undertake teaching outside the operating room. Anaesthesia has expanded to include other services which include Intensive Care, Acute and Chronic Pain Services, Malignant Hyperthermia Diagnostic Services, and a Pre-admission Unit. Anaesthetists have developed many skills which are valuable to physicians, regardless of their discipline. They have become specialists in applied physiology, pharmacology and resuscitation of acutely traumatized patients. The importance of imparting these skills and knowledge to medical students has been realized by those responsible for medical school curricula. Accreditation bodies are demanding that anaesthetists teach medical students.

When the new curriculum, founded on problem-based learning, was adopted in the Faculty of Medicine at the University of Ottawa, anaesthesia was given responsibilities in the program. Each student must spend two weeks in an anaesthesia rotation and many anaesthetists participate in small group sessions. Dr. Patrick Sullivan found that an anaesthesia manual, which would meet the needs of medical students submerged in a new curriculum, was not available. The manual he and his co-authors have written covers all of the important material a medical student must and should know. It is best taught by anaesthetists because it falls almost exclusively in their domain. The organization of the manual makes it essential reading for students rotating through anaesthesia who want to optimize their brief exposure to anaesthesia, which has so much to offer.

J. Earl Wynands, M.D.
Professor and Chairman
Department of Anaesthesia
University of Ottawa

Table of Contents

CHAPTER 1

Anaesthesia Rotational Objectives

There are **six specific knowledge and skills objectives*** for the two week anaesthesia rotation:

1. **To become aware of anaesthetic considerations in the preoperative evaluation and preparation of the patient.**

This will be accomplished by conducting several preoperative assessments, including:

a. Taking and recording a pertinent history.
b. Performing an appropriate physical examination, including assessment of the airway, the respiratory and cardiovascular systems, and other systems as indicated.
c. Reviewing relevant laboratory data.
d. Preparing a problem list and assigning appropriate ASA physical status.
e. Prescribing appropriate premedication, including continuing relevant current medications, and demonstrating knowledge of the principles of managing specific medications (eg. insulin, anticoagulants).

2. **To learn appropriate airway and ventilatory management.**

The student will demonstrate proper airway and ventilatory management of the unconscious patient by:

a. Describing and identifying basic oropharyngeal and laryngotracheal anatomy.
b. Describing the indications, benefits and risks of airway management by mask and endotracheal intubation.
c. Identifying and stating appropriate sizes of masks, oral and nasal airways, laryngoscope blades and endotracheal tubes.
d. Identifying and overcoming upper airway obstruction with mask ventilation using various masks, oral and nasal airways, jaw thrust and or chin lift maneuvers.
e. Successfully preparing appropriate equipment, positioning and intubating several patients with minimal supervisor intervention.
f. Correctly identifying within 30 seconds those patients in whom endotracheal intubation was not successful.
g. Recognizing and discussing the need for controlled ventilation using physical signs, cardiovascular parameters, respiratory measurements, and/or arterial blood gases.

h.   Discussing the various methods of monitoring the adequacy of ventilation.
i.   Prescribing appropriate parameters for mechanical ventilation.
j.   Describing and identifying criteria for extubation.

3.   **To acquire skills necessary to prescribe and conduct appropriate fluid and blood component therapy, including establishing vascular access.**

This will be demonstrated by:
a.   Identifying common sites for venous access.
b.   Demonstrating skill at establishing venous access by:
     - using sterile technique.
     - Successfully inserting several peripheral catheters of various calibres.
     - Protecting the venipuncture site and immobilizing the catheter.
c.   Describing the indications and complications of central venous access.
d.   Prescribing perioperative fluid and electrolyte replacement, taking into account such factors as NPO status, preoperative bowel prep, NG suction, fever, blood losses, and third space losses.
e.   Discussing perioperative indications for blood administration, and learning rational use of blood products, and the potential complications of blood product administration.
f.   Correctly interpreting data from the following monitors of volume status:

- examination of the patient.
- pulse and blood pressure.
- urine output.
- invasive monitoring (CVP, PCWP, Arterial pressure waveforms, cardiac output).

4.   **To learn local anaesthetic pharmacology appropriate to general medicine by:**

a.   Classifying commonly used agents according to amide and ester linkage.
b.   Listing commonly used local anaesthetics for:
     - topical use
     - local infiltration
     - peripheral nerve blocks
     - iv (Bier's) block
     - epidural anaesthesia
     - spinal anaesthesia
c.   Listing acceptable doses of at least two agents used for topical and local infiltration anaesthesia.
d.   Describing the diagnostic criteria for, and management of:
     - local anesthetic toxicity.
     - inadvertent intravascular injection of local anaesthetic.
     - allergic reaction to a local anaesthetic.

5.   **To understand the management of pain in the peripartum period and the initiation of neonatal resuscitation.**

This will be demonstrated by:
a.   Discussing indications, contraindications and adverse effects of various modes of obstetrical pain relief.

- mask analgesia with nitrous oxide and/or volatile anaesthetic agents.
- narcotic analgesia (im, or iv).
- epidural anaesthesia.
- spinal anaesthesia.

b. The student will develop skills in assessment and management of the healthy newborn by:
- administering oxygen by mask.
- performing oropharyngeal and nasopharyngeal suction.
- performing an initial physical examination.
- assigning Apgar Scores.
- recognizing newborn distress.

c. The student will be able to describe therapeutic steps necessary to begin neonatal resuscitation.

6. **To understand the principles of acute and chronic pain management.**

This will be achieved through the provided reading material in the anaesthesia manual, a pain clinic rotation, and a discussion of modalities for acute pain management including:

a. iv narcotic infusions.
b. non-narcotic analgesics.
c. iv and epidural PCA (patient controlled analgesia).
d. peripheral nerve blocks.

Reading material in the anaesthesia manual and discussion of the diagnosis and management of common chronic pain syndromes will focus on:

a. Reflex sympathetic dystrophy.
b. Fibrositis.

c. Chronic low back pain.
d. Post herpetic neuralgia.
e. Cancer pain.

ANAESTHESIA CURRICULUM: KNOWLEDGE/SKILLS/ATTITUDE

Knowledge:

The following topics will be covered either in the manual, or in seminar format and problem solving sessions during the 12-week surgical - anaesthesia rotation.

Preoperative evaluation and preparation.
Anaesthetic - Surgical risk assessment.
Hypoxia.
Oxygen Therapy.
Intubation-indications/complications.
Principles of mechanical ventilation.
Shock.
Fluid Therapy.
Blood component therapy.
Acute and Chronic Pain management.
Obstetrical anaesthesia-analgesia.
Basic neonatal resuscitation.

Skills:

1. Airway maintenance maneuvers in the unconscious patient.
2. Artificial airway insertion.
3. Mask ventilation.
4. Endotracheal intubation and extubation.
5. Spontaneous, manual, and controlled modes of ventilation.
6. Venous cannulation.
7. Prescription, identification and administration of blood components, including equipment assembly.[tt]
8. Arterial blood gas sampling.[tt]

9. Spinal anaesthesia
   (Lumbar puncture).[tt]
10. Nasogastric tube insertion.[tt]

[tt] Skills number 1 to 6 must be achieved during the rotation. Students may acquire skills number 7 to 10 depending on clinical opportunity and the students' interest level.

Attitude:

We hope that your two-week rotation will stimulate a thirst for knowledge and understanding of the fascinating physiology and pharmacology that occurs in the patient undergoing surgery. Anaesthesia is a somewhat unnatural if not magical state. It is normal to feel technically challenged during your rotation as you acquire vascular access and airway management skills. Each of you can expect to experience (as all doctors have), a humbling but hopefully rewarding, technical learning curve. You should be aware of your difficulties, your response to them, and the response of your patient and other medical personnel to your difficulties. We ask that your eyes and senses not be clouded by technical monitors, but rather be open to the overall care of the patient. We demand a commitment of excellence in your care and concern for the well-being of the patient and their family. We expect punctuality and honesty as a basis of good medicine.

While students may view anaesthesia as a specialty with limited patient contact, they should ensure that opportunities for communication with the patient and family do not slip by. Fact-gathering encounters do not have to be devoid of reassurance, kindness or a comforting touch. We expect both positive and negative experiences during your rotation to be discussed openly with us, to ensure the best possible rotation for future students.

Resources:

Our University of Ottawa Anaesthesia Manual will be distributed to all students, and will be used as the basic reference text for the rotation. Additional reference material will be available in each hospital's anaesthesia library.

Topics covered in this manual have been classified as either *must know, should know*, or *may know* material. Material designated as *must know* will be identified by two asterisks (**), and will have a greater emphasis in content and weighting in the multiple choice, short answer, and OSCE questions at the end of the surgical anaesthesia rotation. Material assigned to the *should know* portion of each chapter will be identified by one asterisk (*). All other topics covered in the manual provide a general background for the student during their anaesthesia rotation, and are topics which the student *may know*. A passing grade can be achieved with a good comprehension of the *must know* material, while an honours mark may be awarded to students correctly answering material covered in the *should know* and *may know* sections of the manual.

A computerized anaesthesia simulator will be available as an option during the students rotation. (The simulator includes models of pharmacology, pharmacokinetics, critical incidents, as well as cardiovascular and respiratory physiology).

The hospitals' anaesthesia library and main libraries will be available for reference during the rotation.

Notes:

Evaluation:

The rotation evaluation will be based on four components.

I.   Participation during problem solving sessions.

II. One or more examinations using a multiple choice format, short answer examination format, or OSCE examination.

III. A clinical profile record.

IV. A review of the anaesthesia simulator problems (optional).

CHAPTER 2

Anaesthesia Overview

Modern general anaesthesia is based on the ability to provide adequate analgesia and amnesia during surgical procedures. Neuromuscular-blocking drugs may be utilized to facilitate surgical exposure by providing profound muscle relaxation. The anaesthesiologist attempts to achieve both analgesia and amnesia, with or without muscle relaxation, while maintaining the patient's normal physiological functions. The challenge in anaesthesia is to maintain a balance between the stress of the surgical procedure and the cardiorespiratory depressant effects of deepening levels of anaesthesia (figure 2.1). The anaesthes-

iologist uses both skills in clinical examination and a host of technical monitors to provide ongoing feedback on the patient's physiological status and anaesthetic requirements. Table 2.1 lists options available to the anaesthesiologist for providing analgesia, amnesia and muscle relaxation.

A state of general anaesthesia may be induced with the injection of anaesthetic drugs, or by the inhalation of a mixture of anaesthetic vapours (figure 2.1). With general anaesthesia, muscle relaxants may be used to facilitate both tracheal intubation and muscle relaxation.

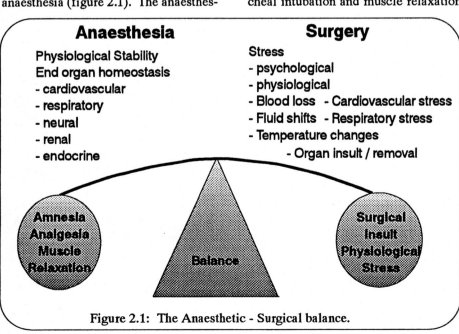

Figure 2.1: The Anaesthetic - Surgical balance.

Muscle relaxants are frequently used to facilitate surgical access, and are essential for thoracic and abdominal operations. As muscle relaxants have no effect on the state of consciousness, additional anaesthetic medications must be given to ensure both amnesia and analgesia. The use of muscle relaxants avoids the need for excessive amounts of other anaesthetic agents that would otherwise be required to achieve the same degree of muscle relaxation. Because muscle relaxants also affect the muscles of respiration, positive pressure ventilation is frequently used to maintain normal minute ventilation when they are given. When muscle relaxants are not used, the patient may be allowed to spontaneously inhale anaesthetic vapours to maintain the anaesthetic state. If efforts at spontaneous ventilation are inadequate, manually assisted or controlled mechanical ventilation may be used by the anaesthetist. Controlled mechanical ventilation is generally used only when the trachea has been intubated.

Table 2.1: Anaesthetic Options*.

Anaesthetic Options	
Local Anaesthesia Alone.	
Local Anaesthesia with intravenous conscious sedation.	eg. iv Propofol, midazolam, fentanyl and or music for sedation.
Neurolept-analgesia.	Used infrequently. Achieved with high doses of droperidol with a opioid (such as fentanyl) for analgesic supplementation.
Regional Anaesthesia, with or without sedation.	eg. Spinal Anaesthesia Epidural Anaesthesia Brachial Plexus Block Intravenous 'Bier' Block Peripheral Nerve Blocks
General Anaesthesia. (see figure 2.2)	May be combined with regional anaesthesia, peripheral nerve blocks or local anaesthesia.
Others	Acupuncture Biofeedback techniques (Lamaze) Inhalational agents (eg. Entonox = 50:50 mixture of nitrous oxide and oxygen). im, po, iv sedatives, narcotics, neuroleptics, or antiemetics

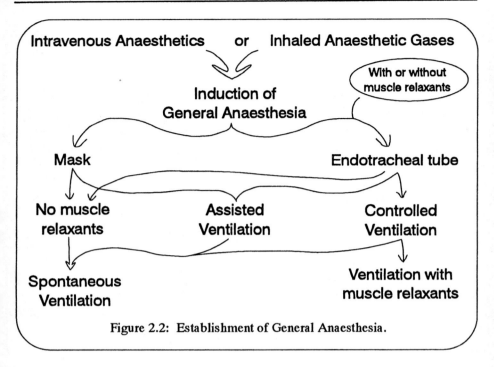

Figure 2.2: Establishment of General Anaesthesia.

Spontaneous and assisted ventilation may be used in conjunction with a tracheal tube, laryngeal mask airway, or simple face mask (figure 2.2).

Modern general anaesthesia uses combinations of medications in an attempt to minimize each drug's side effects, and maximize individual benefits. Hence, rather than using halothane alone to provide anaesthesia for abdominal surgery, the anaesthetist often chooses a series of medications to match the patient's needs. These medications may include opioids to blunt the pain response to surgery, barbiturates to induce the anaesthetic state, and volatile anaesthetic agents such as nitrous oxide and isoflurane to maintain the anaesthetic state. Other common anaesthetic drugs used during general anaesthesia include antiemetics, neuromuscular blocking agents, and neuromuscular antagonists.

CHAPTER 3

Preoperative Evaluation and Risk Assessment

GREG BRYSON M.D., FRCPC AND JOHN B. KITTS M.D., FRCPC

Preoperative assessment is essential for the safety of anaesthesia. Physicians who have had no exposure to the specialty of anaesthesia are ill-equipped to evaluate, prepare, and institute measures to minimize the patient's risk in the perioperative period. This chapter provides a framework for physicians who need to understand their patients' risk of undergoing a surgical procedure, and the measures that can be used to optimize their patients' condition prior to surgery.

Preoperative evaluation serves many purposes. First, it offers the anaesthetist an opportunity to define the patient's medical and surgical problems, and plan the anaesthetic technique. Second, further investigation, consultation, and treatment can be arranged for patients whose condition is not optimal. Finally, the anaesthetist can provide information and reassurance for the patient during this stressful time.

An organized approach to the preoperative evaluation will allow the anaesthetist to perform a focused evaluation of the patient's medical and surgical condition, and to address issues relevant to the safe and effective performance of surgery. The preoperative evaluation does not replace the role of the primary care provider, and should not be used to address issues that are not relevant to the performance of anaesthesia and surgery.

The preoperative visit should include the following steps:

I. Problem Identification
II. Risk Assessment
III. Preoperative Preparation
IV. Plan of Anaesthetic Technique

I. PROBLEM IDENTIFICATION**

Identification of the problems a patient brings to the operating room is one of the most vital, yet easily neglected, components of the perioperative management of the surgical patient. A system-oriented approach to the patient is helpful in completing a thorough preoperative assessment. As is the case elsewhere in medicine, the preoperative evaluation should progress through history (including a review of the patient's chart), physical examination, and laboratory investigation.

Anaesthetic drugs and techniques have profound effects on human physiology. Hence, a focused review of all major organ systems should be completed prior to surgery. The anaesthetist pays special attention to symptoms and disease related to the cardiovascular, respiratory, and neuromuscular systems as they will directly manipulate these systems during surgery. Because one of the goals of the preoperative evaluation is to ensure that the patient is in the *best* (or optimal) *condition*, it is important not only to identify symptoms, but also to document their severity and to determine their stability or progress. Patients with unstable symptoms should be postponed for optimization prior to elective surgery.

Cardiovascular:

Patients with *ischemic heart disease* are at risk for myocardial ischaemia or infarction in the perioperative period. A thorough history should ascertain whether angina is new or has recently changed from a previously stable pattern. A description of the patient's exercise tolerance must also be included. Patients with a history of a recent myocardial infarction (< 6 months) or unstable angina are poor surgical candidates, with a high risk of significant morbidity or mortality.

Assessment of cardiac risk is discussed later in this chapter. As many anaesthetic agents are also myocardial depressants, a history of *congestive heart failure* or *cardiomyopathy* should

be directly sought. *Valvular heart disease* presents a special set of concerns to the anaesthetist. This includes unfavourable and even dangerous alterations in haemodynamics brought on by the anaesthesia, particularly major regional techniques (see chapter 15: Local and regional anaesthetics). Consider the risk of subacute bacterial endocarditis (SBE) in these patients.

Although less common with new anaesthetic drugs, *arrhythmias* are frequently seen in the operating room. In the preoperative visit, identify a past history of arrhythmia or symptoms suggesting the need for a pacemaker. The patient with *hypertension* will require special attention to perioperative antihypertensive therapy and fluid and electrolyte balance.

Respirology:

Cigarette smoke has several adverse effects, including alteration of mucus secretion, clearance, and decrease in small airway calibre. It also may alter the immune response. The chronic smoker should be encouraged to abstain from smoking for at least 8 weeks prior to the operation,[1] but stopping smoking for even 24 hours may produce benefits in cardiovascular physiology[2] and carboxyhemoglobin levels.

Patients with chronic *obstructive pulmonary disease (COPD)* are at increased risk of perioperative respiratory complications. Anaesthesia, surgery and postoperative analgesia all predispose the patient with COPD to respiratory depression, atelectasis, retained secretions, pneumonia and respiratory insufficiency or failure. The patient with *asthma* is at particular risk as manipulation of the airway and cold dry anaesthetic gases are potent triggers of intraoperative bronchospasm. Determine the presence of cough and the colour and amount of sputum. Ensure that there is no acute upper respiratory infection.

The patient's exercise capacity should be evaluated by asking questions such as how they manage around stairs at home, and walking to local stores. Are they able to walk several blocks comfortably at a normal pace? Do they avoid stairs? If they routinely uses stairwells, how many flights are they able to complete? Do they have to rest in the stairwell? Is this the result of fatigue, shortness of breath, or chest pain?

Restrictive lung disease will be worsened by upper abdominal or thoracic surgery, and place the patient at increased risk for perioperative failure. Any disease process which leads to an *altered control of breathing* (obstructive sleep apnea, CNS disorders, etc.) may lead to profound respiratory depression from the drugs used in the perioperative period, and may require postoperative monitoring in a critical care setting. Potential *airway* problems are of particular concern to the anaesthetist, and must always be evaluated (see chapter 6: Intubation and Anatomy of the Airway).

Neuromuscular:
If the patient has an intracranial lesion, seek early signs and symptoms of *raised intracranial pressure* such as headaches, nausea, vomiting, confusion and papilledema. *Pituitary lesions* may cause endocrine abnormalities. A history of *TIA's* or *CVA's* suggests significant cerebrovascular disease. The anaesthetist should ask the patient about a history of *seizures*, and determine the type, frequency and time of last occurrence. Note any anticonvulsant medications the patient is receiving.

The patient with a history of *spinal cord injury* is at risk for a number of perioperative complications including respiratory failure, arrhythmias, autonomic hyperreflexia, hyperkalemia, pathologic fractures and pressure sores. It is important to document the date and level of the neurological injury, as the incidence of many of these complications are dependent on such variables. Patients with *lower motor neuron lesions* of any kind are at risk for unusual responses to anaesthetic drugs (see chapter 12: Muscle Relaxants - Succinylcholine), and regional anaesthesia should be considered only after careful documentation of the patient's nerve deficits.

Disorders of the *neuromuscular junction* such as myasthenia gravis, myasthenic syndrome, etc., will cause unpredictable responses to neuromuscular-blocking drugs. Lastly, patients with *muscular dystrophies* and underlying myopathies are known to have both an increased association with malignant hyperthermia and an increased risk of postoperative respiratory failure (see chapter 24: Uncommon Anaesthetic Complications - Malignant Hyperthermia).

Endocrine:

Patients with *diabetes mellitus* require careful management in the perioperative period, as the stress of surgery and perioperative fasting can cause marked swings in blood glucose. Diabetics frequently have widespread end organ damage involving the cardiovascular, nervous and renal systems.

Patients with *thyroid disease* may experience difficulties under anaesthesia. Profound hypothyroidism is associated with myocardial depression and exaggerated responses to sedative medications. Hyperthyroid patients are at risk for perioperative thyroid storm. Thyroid goitres may compress the airway and involve the recurrent laryngeal nerve leading to vocal cord palsy. These place the patient at risk for airway obstruction.

Patients with *phaeochromocytoma* are particularly challenging for the anaesthetist, surgeon, and internist involved in their care. These patients are at risk for extreme swings in blood pressure and heart rate in the perioperative period, and require intensive preoperative therapy with adrenergic blocking drugs. Patients at risk for *adrenal suppression* (history of exogenous steroid therapy) may not be able to increase their own corticosteroid production to match the imposed stress of surgery. The incidence of adrenal suppression is not predictable, and depends on the potency and frequency of steroid dose and on the length of steroid therapy. As a general rule, corticosteroid supplementation is provided for patients who have required steroids for more than one week in the last six months.

GI-Hepatic:

Patients with *hepatic disease* frequently present problems with fluid and electrolyte imbalance, coagulopathies and altered drug metabolism. Patients with *gastroesophageal reflux* (GER), as well as those at risk for GER, are prone to regurgitation of gastric contents and aspiration pneumonitis during the perioperative period (see chapters 9 & 24: Rapid Sequence Induction & Unusual Anaesthetic Complications - Aspiration Pneumonitis). These patients should receive anti-reflux prophylaxis preoperatively.

Renal:

Disorders of *fluid and electrolyte balance* are common in the perioperative period, and management of any possible electrolyte deficiency or excess may be part of the anaesthetic management of the patient. Generally all fluid and electrolyte disorders should be corrected prior to elective surgery.

Patients with *renal failure*, both acute and chronic, frequent the OR. The anaesthetist must be prepared to deal with their fluid and electrolyte disorders, dialysis requirements and altered drug metabolism. Pay careful attention to the patient's dialysis schedule, as important changes in blood volume and serum potassium levels occur pre- and post-dialysis. If possible, plan elective surgery so that the patient receives dialysis either the night before surgery, or on the morning of surgery. Patients with renal insufficiency are at risk for deterioration of their renal function, and careful attention must be paid to their fluid and haemodynamic management in the perioperative period.

Haematologic:

Anemias of a variety of causes are common in the patient undergoing surgery. A minimum haemoglobin level of 100 gm/L was traditionally required before a patient could undergo elective surgery. The dogma regarding an adequate haemoglobin level has held less sway in recent years. Now the "transfusion trigger" must be individualized to the patient, bearing in mind the chronicity of the anemia, the likelihood of perioperative blood loss, and the patient's co-existent disease (see chapter 20).

Coagulopathies involving clotting factors and platelets, both congenital and acquired, require careful management. Patients with a bleeding tendency are generally poor candidates for major regional anaesthesia and management must be individualized, depending on the nature of the bleeding problem, the proposed surgery, and the patient's medical condition.

The Elderly:

The elderly have a higher incidence of age-related coexisting disease as well as both diminished organ function and organ reserve. The result is that elderly patients are generally recognized to be in a higher perioperative risk group. Perioperative morbidity and mortality are related to the extent of coexisting disease rather than the patient's age alone. Elderly patients should not be refused elective surgery on the basis of their age alone. However, every attempt must be made in adequately diagnosing and treating coexisting disease preoperatively. The risk of deferring surgery must be balanced against the potential for the patient returning on an emergency basis.

Emergency surgery in the elderly patient may lead to a four- to twenty-fold increase in perioperative mortality. Delay in presentation and inadequate time for optimizing coexisting disease place an increased burden on a patient lacking the physiological reserve to tolerate major stress and surgery.

Medications and Allergies:

A detailed list of the patients' medications and allergies is an essential part of the preoperative assessment. Particular attention should be paid to cardiovascular and respiratory medications, narcotic analgesics, and drugs known to have significant side effects or drug interactions.

As a general rule, all cardiac and pulmonary medications and most other necessary medications should be taken with sips of water at the usual time, up to and including the day of surgery. Possible exceptions to this include coumadin, ASA and NSAID's, insulin (adjustment of the dose is needed on the day of surgery), oral hypogylcemics and antidepressants. Pay special attention to patients receiving monoamine oxidase (MAO) inhibitors and amiodarone.

Question patients with allergies to drugs carefully on the nature of the reaction and the circumstances under which it occurred. Many "allergies" are simply anticipated drug side effects such as nausea and vomiting, or adrenaline absorption from local anaesthetic agents. True allergies to anaesthetics are unusual, but when present, can be fatal.

Prior Anaesthetics:

The patient undergoing anaesthesia and surgery should be carefully questioned on their response to previous anaesthetics and a family history of problems with anaesthesia. Investigate any complication or adverse reaction to prior anaesthetics. Document the type of problem, as well as its management and outcome. In the case of serious perioperative events, consult the old chart to complete the history. Seek a family history of adverse anaesthetic experience. Malignant hyperthermia and plasma cholinesterase deficiency are two hereditary disorders that manifest under anaesthesia (see chapter 24: Unusual Anaesthetic Complications).

Problems related to Surgery:

Information about the patient's general medical condition and anticipated intraoperative problems can be gained from an evaluation of the proposed surgery. Careful consideration of the surgical procedure will reveal the likelihood of significant blood or third space loss, cardiorespiratory compromise, and/or unusual positioning requirements (prone, lateral, lithotomy, etc.). This information will be useful in planning venous access, monitoring, and anaesthetic technique.

Physical Examination:

The physical examination should focus on evaluation of the airway, the cardiovascular system, the respiratory system, and any other systems identified as having symptoms or disease from the history.

General:

A general assessment of the patient's physical and mental status is performed. Note whether the patient is alert, calm, and cooperative, or unusually anxious about their scheduled procedure. Is the patient young and physically fit, or elderly incoherent, emaciated and confined to bed? Such obvious differences will dictate the extent and intensity of the examination and the time required to listen to the patient's concerns and provide reassurance. The patient's mental status also influences the type and amount of preoperative medication required (if any), and may influence the type of anaesthetic technique used (eg. general vs. regional).

Upper airway:

Examination of the upper airway must be performed on all patients. Identify and document any loose teeth, capped teeth, or bridges. The patient should be asked to open their mouth as widely as possible, in order to assess temporal mandibular joint mobility, and allow visualization of the soft palate, uvula, pharyngeal arches and posterior pharynx. The thyromental distance (the distance from the mentum (lower border of the chin) to the thyroid notch, the mobility of the C-spine in both flexion and extension, as well as the position of the trachea should all be assessed, as each of these have implications with respect to the ease of intubation.

Assessment of the upper airway must include evaluation of the range of motion of the neck, as well as mouth opening, dentition, and thryromental distance. The adequacy of visualization of the hypopharyngeal structures is used as an indicator of potential difficulty with direct laryngoscopy. A hypopharyngeal class is assigned in an attempt to quantify the degree of difficulty that will be encountered during direct laryngoscopy.[3,4] (See Chapter 6: Anatomy and Assessment of the Airway).

Lower airway:
Assess the respiratory rate. Note the shape of the thoracic cage, and whether or not the patient is relying on their accessory muscles (e.g., the barrel shaped bronchitic patient vs. the pink emphysemic puffer). Auscultate the chest for audible rhonchi on quiet and forced expiration, and identify the presence or absence of rales. Note the presence or absence of cyanosis and clubbing.

Cardiovascular:
Assess the heart rate, rhythm and blood pressure. Identify the location of the apical impulse, and whether it is abnormally displaced. Assess the level of the JVP, and identify the presence or absence of peripheral edema. Identify the first and second heart sounds and listen for the presence of heart murmurs, or a third or fourth heart sound.

Anticipate any special invasive procedures, and assess the anatomy for arterial line insertion, central vein cannulation, intravenous access, and sites for major regional anaesthetic techniques (eg. spinal, epidural, or brachial plexus blocks).

Again, the state of health of the patient will dictate the intensity of the examination required. The healthy 20-year-old male undergoing an arthroscopy, requires a much more abbreviated history, physical examination and chart review when compared to the elderly patient undergoing a major abdominal procedure.

Laboratory Testing:
Obtain preoperative laboratory testing only if indicated from the preoperative history and physical examination. In September 1993, the Public Hospital's Act in Ontario was amended so that mandatory haemoglobin and urine analysis were no longer required prior to surgery. Perform these tests and all other preoperative tests, however, where indicated by the medical status of the patient, or if the patient is considered in a population at risk for a specific problem. "Routine or standing" preoperative tests should be discouraged.

Do a CBC for patients in whom there is significant blood loss anticipated, suspected haematological disorder (eg. anaemia, thalassaemia, sickle cell disease), or recent chemotherapy. Patients on antihypertensive medications, including diuretics, chemotherapy, renal disease, adrenal or thyroid disorders, must have electrolytes evaluated preoperatively. Obtain an electrocardiogram (ECG) for patients over 50 years of age, or those who have a history of cardiac disease, hypertension, peripheral vascular disease, diabetes mellitus, renal, thyroid or metabolic disease. Request chest X-rays prior to cardio-thoracic procedures and for patients with debilitating COPD, asthma, or a change in respiratory symptoms in the past six months. Perform urine analysis for patients with diabetes mellitus, renal disease or recent urinary tract infection.

II: RISK ASSESSMENT

There are three components that must be considered when evaluating peri-operative risk: the patient's medical condition preoperatively, the extent of the surgical procedure, and the risk from the anaesthetic. In general, the major contribution to increased risk is that of the patient's health prior to the procedure and the magnitude of the surgery. However, patients presenting for surgery often have more fear about their anaesthetic than the surgery itself. Fortunately, anaesthesia-related morbidity and mortality is rare, but unfortunately, not absent. This does, however, create its own problems. The combination of infrequent but serious events has led one author to state that "Perhaps the most insidious hazard of anaesthesia is its relative safety."[5]

Anaesthetic Mortality:

The wide variety of surgical procedures and anaesthetic techniques, combined with the diversity of a patient's coexisting surgical and medical illnesses, produce a number of risk factors that contribute to overall outcome, and make generalized statements about risk difficult. Specific predictions for a single patient's outcome is virtually impossible, and the complexity of this issue has made research studies addressing outcome very difficult. Nevertheless, several studies attempting to determine anaesthesia mortality and morbidity have been completed.[6-12] It is difficult to separate the contributions of anaesthesia and surgery to morbidity and mortality, as patients rarely receive an anaesthetic without undergoing a surgical procedure. Table 3.1 summarizes several studies which have attempted to determine the risk of mortality due solely to anaesthesia.

Studies on perioperative mortality have yielded differing results. Differences in the definition of outcome variables, study design, and the duration of follow-up make these results difficult to compare. When reviewed critically, these studies suggest that the often quoted number for overall risk of primary anaesthetic mortality for all patients undergoing all types of surgery is approximately 1:10,000.

The question to which anaesthetists and the patient need the answer is: "What is the risk of a particular procedure in a patient with a given medical status receiving a specific anaesthetic technique?" Numerous investigators have attempted to address this very complex question. Most of the work, however, addresses the operative risk according to the patient's preoperative medical status.

Perioperative Risk Assessment:

Perhaps the oldest and simplest method for risk assessment is the American

Author	Country	Year	No. in study	Incidence of Primary Anaesthetic Mortality
Turnbull[6]	Canada	1980	195,232	1:5,138
Hovi-Vivander[7]	Finland	1980	338,934	1:5,059
Lunn & Mushin[8]	United Kingdom	1982	108,000	1:10,000
Keenan & Boyen[9]	United States	1985	163,240	1:10,000
Tiret[10]	France	1986	198,103	1:13,207
Holland[11]	Australia	1987	550,000	1:26,000
Buck[12]	United Kingdom	1987	500,000	1:185,000

Table 3.1: Estimates of Primary Anaesthetic Mortality

Society of Anesthesiology (ASA) physical status (table 3.2). The ASA physical status classification system was originally proposed in 1941, and revised by Dripps in 1961[13] to provide a uniform assessment of a patient's preoperative physical condition.

As this system is simple, easy to use, and requires no laboratory investigations, it has now been widely accepted as the standard means of preoperative patient classification. Although developed as a tool for classifying a patient's physical condition, the ASA physical status has been used to stratify patient risk. While open to significant criticism because of its vague categories and inconsistencies in its application, the ASA physical status classification has been shown to correlate with perioperative mortality.[14-17]

Category	Description
I	Healthy patient.
II	Mild systemic disease - no functional limitation.
III	Severe systemic disease - definite functional limitation.
IV	Severe systemic disease - a constant threat to life.
V	Moribund patient - not expected to survive with or without an operation for 24 hours.
E	A suffix E is added to denote an emergency procedure.

Table 3.2: ASA Physical Status Classification.

Operative Mortality (percent)				
ASA Class	Vercanti[14] 1970	Marx[15] 1973	Cohen[16] 1986	Forrest[17] 1990
I	.07	.06	.07	.00
II	.24	.40	.20	.04
III	1.43	4.3	1.15	.59
IV	7.46	23.4	7.66	7.95
V	9.38	50.7	-----	-----

Table 3.3: ASA Physical Status vs. Operative Mortality (%).

Examples of the ASA classification:

ASA 1: Healthy patient, no medical problems.
ASA 2: Controlled hypertension.
ASA 3: Emphysema.
ASA 4: Unstable angina.
ASA 5E: Ruptured abdominal aortic aneurysm in shock, undergoing emergency surgery.

Cardiac Risk:
Several perioperative risk studies have attempted to assess which perioperative cardiac risk factors are important. Ischaemic heart disease has received the most attention because mortality from a perioperative myocardial infarction approaches 50%.

In 1977 Goldman published a multifactorial risk index for cardiac patients undergoing non-cardiac procedures[18] (table 3.4). This study, involving 1001 patients, identified, by multivariate analysis, nine potential risk factors that predicted life-threatening cardiac complications. A scoring system weighted these factors in their ability to predict adverse cardiac outcome.

From these data, Goldman suggested that patients with a score greater than 25 be considered only for life-saving procedures. Patients scoring 13-25 were advised to have preoperative medical consultations to lower their morbidity and mortality. Certainly, delaying surgery until the patient is more stable can significantly reduce the cardiac risk index. Waiting for 6 months after a

Risk Factor	Points
Third heart sound or elevated JVP	11
MI within 6 months of surgery	10
Rhythm other than sinus or PAC's	7
> 5 PVC's per minute	7
Age > 70	5
Emergency procedure	4
Abdominal, thoracic, or aortic surgery	3
Important Aortic stenosis	3
Poor medical status	3

Table 3.4: Goldman's Cardiac Risk Index

Variable	Points
MI < 6 months pre-op	10
MI > 6 months pre-op	5
CCS Class 4 angina	20
CCS Class 3 angina	10
Unstable angina < 3 months pre-op	10
Pulmonary edema < 1 week pre-op	10
Pulmonary edema ever	5
Critical aortic stenosis	20
Rhythm other than sinus	5
> 5 PVC's per minute	5
Poor medial status	5
Age > 70 years	5
Emergency procedure	10

Table 3.5: Detsky's Multifactorial Index

myocardial infarct, delaying emergency procedures (if feasible) and improving a patient's poor medical status all significantly decrease the risk.

The Goldman index has high specificity but low sensitivity when predicting risk. Patients with scores of 13 or greater should arouse suspicion. A low score correlates with a low probability of poor outcome. In an attempt to improve the sensitivity of Goldman's index, Detsky[19] modified Goldman's criteria to include a wider range of cardiac illness (table 3.5). Detsky also recognized that not all surgery carries the same risk, and factored in the surgical procedures for the pretest probability of inducing significant cardiac complications (table 3.6).[19]

Using likelihood ratios, Detsky was able to construct a nomogram relating the pretest probability of cardiac morbidity for the surgical procedure to the patient's risk score. This generates an overall prediction of the risk of major cardiac morbidity or mortality for a patient of a certain medical status undergoing a specific procedure. Although Detsky's risk index is a better

Surgery	% Cardiac Complications
Vascular	13.2
Orthopaedic	13.6
Thoracic - Abdominal	8.0
Head & Neck	2.6
Minor (TURP, Hernia,...)	1.6

Table 3.6: Detsky's Pretest Probability For Type of Surgery

predictor of cardiac outcome than Goldman's, it still has limitations. However, a review of the risk factors described in both these studies alerts the anaesthetist to symptoms or signs of significant disease that may contribute to adverse outcome.

Both Goldman and Detsky identified recent myocardial infarction as a risk factor for perioperative cardiac morbidity. The perioperative period is characterized by haemodynamic changes, alterations in ventilation, fluid and electrolyte shifts, and changes in coagulation, all of which place the patient with underlying cardiac illness at significant risk of infarction. Several important studies have been conducted over the past 20 years in an attempt to identify the likelihood of perioperative reinfarction in patients with a recent MI.[20-22] The goal of these studies was to determine the safest time interval following an MI to proceed with elective surgery, and to direct attention to appropriate perioperative monitoring and care (Table 3.7).

In Rao's study, patients were managed with invasive haemodynamic monitoring and aggressive therapy in an intensive care unit (ICU) setting for 72 hours following surgery. Cumulatively, these studies suggest considerable benefit in delaying elective surgery for a period of 6 months following a myocardial infarction. Before six months, invasive monitoring and aggressive postoperative management, appear essential, for those patients in whom surgery must be performed.

III: PREOPERATIVE PREPARATION*

Premedication: (see also chapter 4)
Anaesthetic indications: The preanaesthetic visit should be designed to alleviate patient anxiety and apprehension about the proposed surgery. However, a benzodiazepine such as diazepam or lorazepam is also frequently administered orally 1 - 2 hours preoperatively. This may provide sedation, relieve anxiety, and provide a degree of amnesia for the events immediately preceding the operation.

Patients at risk for GE reflux should receive anti-reflux prophylaxis. This is

Time from infarction to Surgery	Tarhan20 (1972)	Steen21 (1978)	Rao22 (1983)
0 - 3 months	37%	27%	5.8%
3 - 6 months	16%	11%	2.3%
Greater than 6 months	5.6%	4.1%	1.5%

Table 3.7: Comparison of Perioperative Reinfarction Rates (%).

usually achieved with ranitidine 150 - 300 mg p.o. 2 hours pre-operatively. Other agents such as metoclopramide may be added to promote gastric emptying. Sodium citrate is an effective nonparticulate antacid that may also be used alone or in conjunction with ranitidine.

Surgical indications: According to the American Heart Association Guidelines, appropriate antibiotic prophylaxis must be administered for patients at risk for the development of infective endocarditis.[23] These include patients for whom a bacteremia is likely to occur as a result of respiratory tract, genitourinary, or gastrointestinal tract interventions. Some patients are at high risk for the development of postoperative deep vein thrombosis (DVT). Prophylactic measures should be used and include low-dose heparin, intermittent calf compression, or coumadin. Patients who are currently receiving steroids and those who have required steroids in the previous six months may require supplemental steroids because of adrenal suppression and a blunted response to stress.

Co-existing Disease Indications: All important medications should be continued on the day of surgery. These can be taken orally with sips of water. Some medications, including insulin, prednisone, coumadin, and bronchodilators, require adjustment of dosage and/or alternate routes of administration. Oral hypoglycemics and antidepressants should not be taken on the day of surgery. It is no longer mandatory to discontinue MAO inhibitors two weeks preoperatively.

IV: PLANNING THE ANAESTHETIC**

Having identified and evaluated our patient's problems we now ask ourselves five questions.

1.   **Is the patient's condition optimal?**

2.   **Are there any problems which require consultation or special tests?**

(For example: In a patient with poorly controlled angina, a cardiology consult would be appropriate. You may write: *Consult medicine - cardiology. 'Please assess and advise re: optimal perioperative medical management of angina in this patient'*).

3.   **Is there an alternative procedure which may be more appropriate?**

This is especially important to consider in the high risk patient. For example: the placement of a suprapubic catheter may be more appropriate than a transurethral prostatectomy (TURP) in a terminal cancer patient with a recent stroke, congestive heart failure, and obstructive uropathy. Discuss the available options with the staff anaesthetist and the surgeon.

4.   **What are the plans for postoperative management of the patient?**

Options include: Monitoring in the post-anaesthesia care unit (PACU) for an initial period of observation, then either return to ward or discharge home (e.g., daycare patients). Patients with significant underlying diseases or having major procedures may remain in a critical care setting overnight for closer observation (eg. PACU, ICU, CCU). Consideration should be given to which form of pain management is most appropriate for the patient postoperatively.

5. What premedication if any is appropriate?

Finally, we plan our anaesthetic technique (see chapter 2: Anaesthesia Overview). This may be:
1. Local anesthesia with 'standby' monitoring with or without sedation.
2. Regional anesthesia with or without intraoperative sedation.
3. General anesthesia with or without intubation. If an intubation is required the anaesthetist may elect to control the patient's ventilation, or allow them to breath spontaneously. If controlled ventilation is used, the anaesthetist may or may not use muscle relaxants.
4. Combined regional anaesthesia with general anaesthesia.

Discuss with your staff anaesthetist when and why we would choose each of these techniques.

For discussion, let us work through a patient case. We recently gave an anaesthetic to a 50-year-old male for an elective repair of his inguinal hernia. He admitted to smoking one package of cigarettes per day, and has done so for the last 35 years. He has had hypertension for the last six years, and was also found to have NIDDM at the time his hypertension was diagnosed.

Our patient's problem list includes:
1. Elective lower abdominal surgery.
2. Controlled hypertension.
3. NIDDM.
4. Smoking history 35 pack years.
5. Identified risk factors for CAD.

The anaesthetic *history* should include:
1. A brief *history of present illness*. E.g., "Discomfort in groin for 6 months."
2. Current *medications* (including ASA, alcohol, and illicit drugs if appropriate). E.g., "Enalapril 10 mg and glyburide 10 mg daily."
3. *Allergies* and type of reaction. E.g., "Penicillin: hives."
4. Significant *past medical - surgical history*. E.g., "Appendectomy".
5. *Past anaesthetic history.* E.g., "No known problems."
6. *Family history* of any anaesthetic problems. E.g., "No known problems." (see chapter 24).
7. *Functional inquiry* appropriate to the patient, and concentrating on the cardiorespiratory systems. E.g., "Inactive lifestyle, no symptoms of chest pain or coronary ischemia." (See also 9 below re: additional appropriate questions.
8. *NPO status.* E.g., "Nothing to eat or drink since last night."
9. *Specific questions* directed at the identified problem list, attempting to assess the severity of the problem, its associated disability, and the patient's remaining physiological reserve.

Problem: *35 pack year smoker.*

Do you have a cough on most mornings or a "smoker's cough"? (i.e. Chronic bronchitis).
Do you ever wheeze?
Have you ever required medications for your breathing?
Does your breathing limit your physical activity?
What kind of activity would make you short of breath? (A fast walk? One flight of stairs? Two blocks? etc.).

Problem: *Hypertension.*

When were you first aware that you had high blood pressure?
How often is your blood pressure checked?
Has it been well controlled with your medications?
What is your usual blood pressure when you see your family doctor?

Problem: *NIDDM*

How long have you been aware of your diabetes?
How has it affected you? (end organs involved include: eyes, heart, kidneys, peripheral circulation, autonomic and peripheral nerves).
How do you monitor your blood sugar?
Have you ever had to come to the emergency because of your diabetes?

Identified risk factors for CAD include hypertension, smoking history, male gender, age and diabetes.

Appropriate questions concerning his cardiovascular risk factors would include:

Have you ever had a heart attack?
Do you ever get chest pains, or leg cramps with exertion? (Angina, claudication).
How often? What relieves them? What are they like?
Do you ever wake up at night short of breath? (PND).
Are you able to sleep with the head of the bed flat? (Orthopnea)

Additional appropriate questions for this patient would include questions regarding gastroesophageal reflux.
Do you ever experience acid reflux from your stomach? How often?

Next, a physical examination as described previously should be performed.

Appropriate laboratory tests for this patient would include a CBC, electrolytes, glucose, and electrocardiogram.

After discussion with the patient and surgeon, a spinal anaesthetic was chosen for this patient. While a general anaesthetic would also be an option, we chose a spinal anaesthetic because we would be able to avoid intubation and its associated sympathetic stimulation (increased heart rate and blood pressure), as well as its potential to trigger airway reflexes resulting in bronchospasm.

References:

1. Warner MA, Offord KP, Warner ME et al. Role of preoperative cessation of smoking and other factors in postoperative pulmonary complications: a blinded prospective study of coronary artery bypass patients. Mayo Clin Proc 64:609, 1989

2. Pierce AC, Jones RM: Smoking and anesthesia: preoperative abstinence and perioperative mortality. Anesthesiology 61:576, 1984

3. Mallampati SR, Gatt SP, Gugino LD, et al: A clinical sign to predict difficult tracheal intubation: A prospective study. Can J Anaesth 32:429, 1985.

4. Samsoon GLT, Young JRB: Difficult tracheal intubation: A retrospective study. Anaesthesia 42:487, 1987.

5. Cooper JB, Newbower RS, Kitz RJ: An analysis of major errors and equipment failures in anaesthesia management: Considerations for prevention and detection. Anesthesiology 60:34, 1984.

6. Turnbull KW, Fancourt-Smith PF, Banting GC: Death within 48 hours of Anaesthesia at the Vancouver General Hospital. Can Anaesth Soc J 27:159, 1980.

7. Hovi-Viander M: Death associated with anaesthesia in Finland. Br J Anaesth 52:483, 1980.

8. Lunn JN, Mushin WW: Mortality associated with anaesthesia. Nuffield Provincial Hospitals Trust, London. 1982.

9. Keenan RL, Boyan CP. Cardiac arrest due to anesthesia: A study of incidence and causes. JAMA 253:2372, 1985.

10. Tiret L, Desmonts JM, Hatton F, et al: Complications associated with anaesthesia - a prospective study in France. Can J Anaesth 33:336, 1986.

11. Holland R. Anaesthetic mortality in New South Wales. Br J Anaesth 59:834, 1987.

12. Buck N, Devlin HB, Lunn JL: Report on the confidential enquiry into perioperative deaths. The Nuffield Provincial Hospitals Trust, London. The King's Fund Publishing House, London. 1987.

13. Dripps RD, Lamont A, Eckenoff JE: The role of anaesthesia in surgical mortality. JAMA 178:261, 1961.

14. Vancanti CJ, VanHouten RJ, Hill RC: A statistical analysis of the relationship of physical status to postoperative mortality in 68,388 cases. Anesth Analg 49:564, 1970.

15. Marx GF, Mateo CV, Orkin LR: Computer analysis of post anaesthetic deaths. Anesthesiology 39:54, 1973.

16. Cohen MM, Duncan PG, Pope WDB, et al: A survey of 112,000 anaesthetics at one teaching hospital (1975-83). Can J Anaesth 33:22, 1986.

17. Forrest JB, et al: Multicenter study of general anesthesia. II. Results. Anesthesiology 72:262, 1990.

18. Goldman L, Caldera DL, Nussbaum SR, et al: Multi-factorial index of cardiac risk in non cardiac surgical procedures. N Engl J Med 297:845, 1977.

19. Detsky AS, Abrams HB, Forbath N, et al: Cardiac assessment for patients undergoing non cardiac surgery: A multifactorial clinical risk index. Arch Intern Med 146:2131, 1986.

20. Tarhan S, Moffitt EA, Taylor WF, et al: Myocardial infarction after general anesthesia. JAMA 220:1451, 1972.

21. Steen PA, Tinker JH, Tarhan S: Myocardial re-infarction after anesthesia and surgery. JAMA 239:2566, 1978.

22. Rao TLK, Jacobs KH, El-Etr AA: Re-infarction following anaesthesia in patients with myocardial infarction. Anesthesiology 59:499, 1983.

23. Dajani AS, Bisno Al, Chung KJ, et al: Prevention of bacterial endocarditis. Recommendations by the American Heart Association. JAMA 264:2919, 1990.

Notes:

Notes:

CHAPTER 4

Premedication

Most patients scheduled for surgery will experience some degree of apprehension. The psychological stress a patient experiences prior to surgery can be more detrimental than the actual physical insult of the surgical procedure. Preoperative anxiety may be caused by many factors. Some of the more common causes include*:

1. The fear of relinquishing control to someone else while under general anaesthesia.
2. The fear of dying during the operation.
3. The fear of experiencing pain postoperatively.
4. The inability to preserve their modesty and dignity during the operation.
5. The fear of separation from family, and loved ones.
6. The fear of discovering a serious problem such as cancer.
7. The fear of surgical mutilation and an altered body image.

It is important that time is taken to answer each patient's questions. If you are unable to answer their questions honestly, then reassure them that their questions are important to you and that, while you may not know the answer, you will speak to the attending staff physician and provide them with an answer. Perhaps the most important part of our preoperative visit is to convey a reassuring, honest and caring attitude.

The patient's desire for sedation prior to a planned surgical procedure is the most common reason for prescribing a preoperative medication. We also prescribe medications preoperatively to avoid potential complications associated with the procedure (e.g., antibiotics to prevent the development of endocarditis in a patient with valvular heart disease), or to continue the patient's current medications for coexisting medical conditions.

Reasons* for prescribing a preoperative medication include:

I. Patient-related reasons:
1. Sedation
2. Amnesia
3. Analgesia
4. Antisialogogue effect (to dry oral secretions)
5. Medications to decrease gastric acidity and gastric volume.
6. To facilitate induction of anaesthesia.

II. Procedure-related reasons:

1. Antibiotic prophylaxis to prevent infective endocarditis in susceptible patients.

2. Gastric prophylaxis (to minimize the risk of gastric aspiration during anaesthesia).
3. Corticosteroid coverage in patients who are immunosuppressed (see chapter 3).
4. To avoid undesired reflexes arising during a procedure (e.g., vagal reflex during eye surgery).
5. Anticholinergic agents to decrease oral secretions and facilitate a planned awake intubation with a fiberoptic bronchoscope.

III. Coexisting Diseases:

1. To continue the patient's own medications for coexisting diseases. (e.g., beta blockers, antihypertensive medications, nitrates, antiparkinsonian medications etc.)
2. To optimize the patients status prior to the procedure. (e.g., bronchodilators, nitroglycerine, beta blockers, antibiotics etc.)

Patients with significant coexisting diseases should be given a reduced amount of preoperative sedative medication. The obese patient does not necessarily require more preoperative medication. It is safer to underestimate the required amount of preoperative medication. Additional medications can be given intravenously as needed when the patient arrives in the operating room. Patients older than 65 years of age should have a reduced drug dosage. Caution should be exercised in prescribing sedatives to patients 75 years of age or older, as they may experience excessive depressant effects from these medications.

Benzodiazepines are the most frequently used class of drugs to achieve sedation, relief of anxiety, and amnesia preoperatively. Diazepam (5 to 15 mg p.o.) may be given with sips of water 1½ to 2 hours preoperatively. Lorazepam (1 to 3 mg) may be given either by the sublingual or oral route. Lorazepam provides excellent amnesia and sedation, but occasionally, patients remain excessively drowsy after the surgery. Alternatively, lorazepam can be reserved for the very anxious patient who is scheduled for afternoon surgery. The rationale of an early morning premedication with lorazepam is to allow the patient to remain calm and relaxed throughout the morning without prolonging the postoperative recovery time. Midazolam (0.07 mg/kg i.m., approximately 5 mg in a young healthy 70 kg adult) provides excellent amnesia, sedation, and anxiolysis when given 1/2 hour preoperatively. Midazolam (as a premedication) is not available at all hospitals. The discomfort of an intramuscular injection and midazolam's associated higher costs have generally made it the third choice of the benzodiazepine class.

Opioids such as morphine and meperidine provide both sedation and analgesia. They are appropriate for patients experiencing pain prior to their surgery, (e.g., fractured extremity awaiting surgery). Morphine has a better sedative effect than meperidine. Troublesome side effects of intramuscular (i.m.) opioids may occur. These include nausea, vomiting, respiratory depression, bradycardia, hypotension, and true allergic reactions. In addition,

Table 4.1: Premedication

Drug / Dose / Route	Class	Comments
Diazepam* (Valium) 5 - 15 mg p.o.	Benzodiazepine	1½ to 2 hours preop. with sips of water. Sedation, amnesia, and anxiolysis. Anticonvulsant (regional anaesthesia). Respiratory depression with high doses.
Lorazepam* (Ativan) 1 - 3 mg p.o. or s.l.	Benzodiazepine	Good amnestic and sedative. Best given early for late case. Occasionally excessive postoperative sedation.
Midazolam (Versed) 0.07 mg/kg i.m. (approx. 5 mg/70 kg)	Benzodiazepine	1/2 to 1 hour preop. Excellent amnestic, sedative, and anxiolytic. Not available in all hospitals.
Morphine* 5 - 15 mg i.m.	Opioid	1 hour preop. Occasional side effects include decreased HR, BP, RR, nausea, biliary spasm and allergic reactions. Better sedative than meperidine.
Meperidine* (Demerol) 50 - 100 mg i.m.	Opioid	1 hour preop. Similar side effects as morphine. Perhaps more nausea, and less biliary spasm.
Atropine* 0.4 - 0.6 mg i.m.	Anticholinergic	1 hour preop. Fair drying agent, often significant tachycardia (HR > 100). Avoid in patients with CAD.
Hyoscine (Scopolamine) 0.2 - 0.4 mg i.m.	Anticholinergic	1 hour preop. Excellent drying agent, confusion in elderly, occas. delirium in young. Good amnestic and antiemetic.
Glycopyrrolate (Robinal) 0.2 - 0.4 mg i.m.	Anticholinergic	Good drying agent for oral secretions, less tachycardia than atropine, no confusion.
Promethazine (Phenergan) 12.5 - 50 mg i.m.	Antihistamine	1 hour preop. Good sedative and antiemetic. Occasional postoperative delirium.

morphine, and to a lesser extent all other opioids, may cause biliary spasm. Opioids should be used with caution in patients with known cholelithiasis.

Drugs with both antiemetic and sedative qualities, are often used in combination with an opioid to avoid nausea and to enhance the sedative effects of the opioid. Promethazine is one such drug (antihistamine - phenothiazine class), and is given in a dose of 12.5 to 50 mg i.m. together with the opioid. Dimenhydrinate (Gravol®) also possesses sedative and antiemetic qualities. It is given in a dose of 12.5 to 50 mg i.m. with the opioid (e.g., *'Demerol 75 mg with gravol 50 mg i.m. in one syringe one hour preoperatively').*

Anticholinergics may be given with morphine or meperidine to avoid the potential opioid-induced bradycardia. An anticholinergic agent may also be used if an awake fiberoptic intubation is planned. The use of an anticholinergic in these patients causes decreased secretions from oral salivary glands, thereby facilitating both absorption of topical anaesthetics and visualization of the airway by a fiberoptic scope. Both hyoscine and atropine cross the blood brain barrier. Hyoscine (0.2 - 0.4 mg i.m.) has been associated with confusion in the elderly and postoperative delirium in young patients. Atropine (0.4 - 0.6 mg i.m.) rarely causes clinical mental confusion. However, it is less effective in drying secretions than hyoscine and causes a greater tachycardia (which is undesirable in the patient with coronary artery disease). Glycopyrrolate (0.2 - 0.4 mg i.m.) is a good drying agent. It does not cross the blood brain barrier and causes less tachycardia than atropine.

Other *special premedications* include: oxygen, antibiotics, steroids, antihistamines, H-2 blockers, beta blockers, calcium channel blockers, nitroglycerine, bronchodilators, antacids, desmopressin, insulin, etc. Ask your staff anaesthesiologist when and why they would prescribe these medications.

General contraindications* to the use of a premedication include:

1. Allergy or hypersensitivity to the drug.
2. Upper airway compromise, or respiratory failure.
3. Hemodynamic instability or shock.
4. Decreased level of consciousness or increased intracranial pressure.
5. Severe liver, renal, or thyroid disease.
6. Obstetrical patients.
7. Elderly or debilitated patients.

Notes:

CHAPTER 5

Getting Started
(A Practical Approach to the OR)

Medical students, beginning their rotation in anaesthesia, will undoubtedly feel unsure of their role and what they ought to do to assist the anaesthesiologist. As anaesthesiologists we observe many operations, however, we recognize that passively watching a procedure does not give us the understanding or skills required to perform it. Accordingly, the more active a role you take in the anaesthetic management of the patient, the more you will get out of the rotation, in terms of understanding, sense of accomplishment, and development of technical skills. Naturally, you should not attempt to perform tasks for which you have little knowledge or supervision. Of all the specialties, anaesthesia is one of the few which can offer intensive one-on-one teaching, and you should try to take as much advantage of this as possible.

What can I do when the patient arrives to the operating room?

Every patient undergoing general, regional, or monitored anaesthesia care requires*:

1. A *safe transfer* from their bed to the operating room table.
2. An *anaesthetic record* removed from the chart and placed on the anaesthesia clipboard. Check to make sure that any information that was missing (eg. Hb, ECG, etc.) at the time of the preoperative visit is now available and on the anaesthetic record.
3. *Monitors attached* including an ECG, blood pressure cuff, and pulse oximeter to start with. (See chapter 10: Monitoring in Anaesthesia).
4. Establish an *intravenous*. Prepare your intravenous equipment before the patient arrives.
5. Record the patients *initial vital signs* on the anaesthesia record.

The above tasks will occupy the first 5 to 10 minutes of your time following the patients arrival in the OR. A *preanaesthetic check list* can be used to ensure that you are ready when the patient arrives to the operating room.

There are many ways anaesthetists ensure that everything is checked and ready to proceed safely with anaesthesia. Whatever system that is used, it should be simple yet comprehensive, and one that will be followed consistently. One such method can be recalled by using the abbreviation *'SAM'*. If you check with *SAM* before you give an anaesthetic, things should proceed smoothly.

What does SAM stand for?

SAM* (really *'SAMMM'*) stands for:

S **Suction** checked and functioning.

A **Airway equipment** checked and prepared. (This includes checking that you have a functioning and backup laryngoscope, an appropriate sized endotracheal tube and stylet, oropharyngeal airways, as well as an oxygen source and manual resuscitation bag).

M **Machine checked.** (see anaesthesia machine checkout procedure and make sure you know how to check your machine. You can go to the operating room before or after scheduled procedures to explore the machine. Ask your staff anaesthetist to go through this procedure with you).

M **Monitors** available and functioning.

M **Medications** prepared and labelled. You should know where the emergency drugs are kept and location of the difficult intubation cart.

You will notice that the last thing that *SAM* has you do is check your medications. If you follow this routine, in this order, you will never put a patient to sleep and then discover, for instance, that their ECG is abnormal, or that a laryngoscope is unavailable.

Anaesthesia Machine Checkout Procedure (Modified from CAS 1989; 36, 6 suppl. 82-7.)

A. Gas Pipelines: Secure connections between terminal units (medical gas outlet) and machine.

B. Anaesthesia Machine:

1. Oxygen and nitrous oxide pipeline pressures should be at 40-60 psi.

2. Check that an adequate amount of oxygen is present in the reserve cylinder on the back of the machine. By turning the cylinder on, the pressure can be read from the pressure gauge on the front of the machine. An oxygen reserve cylinder (E tank) has a full pressure of 2200 psi. The amount in the oxygen tank varies directly with its pressure. Hence, a reading of 1100 psi indicates the tank is half full. A full E tank contains approximately 660 liters of oxygen.

3. Turn the reserve cylinder on the back of the machine off after checking it, to prevent a possible leak from draining the oxygen from the tank.

4. Test that the flowmeters for O2 and N2O are functioning by increasing and decreasing the oxygen and nitrous oxide flows. Ensure that the flowmeter bobbins move freely and do not stick. Turn the nitrous oxide off.

5. The vaporizer should be filled, turned off, and the filling port closed.

6. The oxygen bypass flush valve should release a flush of oxygen when it is activated by pressing the flush button on the front left-hand side of the machine.

7. The oxygen *fail-safe* device should be functioning, and will produce a shrill *Ritchie* whistle if the oxygen pipeline is temporarily disconnected from the wall or ceiling source.

8. Check for the oxygen analyzer which will be located on the respiratory gas monitor or mounted on the machine as a separate unit. It should be turned on and calibrated, if this has not been done recently.
9. The O2 and N2O proportioning device prevents the delivery of less than 30% oxygen, and greater than 70% N2O, and can be tested by varying the O2 and N2O flows through the flowmeter.
10. The common fresh gas outlet located on the front left-hand side of the machine releases anaesthetic gases from the flowmeters, vaporizer and flush valve.

C. Breathing Circuit:
1. The two most common anaesthesia circuits used for adult anaesthesia are the circle circuit and the Bain circuit. An anaesthesia circuit functions to take the anaesthetic gases from the machine to and from the patient. The circle circuit contains a soda lime canister to absorb the exhaled carbon dioxide, an inspiratory and expiratory valve to direct the flow of gases, and light weight corrugated tubing to transport the gases. A sample port near the patient end of the circuit is used for analysis of the respiratory gases. These include inspired and expired oxygen, carbon dioxide, nitrous oxide and volatile anaesthetic gas tensions.
2. Connect the anaesthesia circuit to common fresh gas outlet.
3. Turn the oxygen flowmeter on.
4. Check for fresh gas exiting at the face mask.

5. Pressurize the circuit and check for leaks. (Fill the circuit with fresh gas, occluding the outlet while pressurizing the circuit to 30 cm H2O. The circuit should maintain a pressure of 30 cm H2O with a fresh gas inflow of less than one liter per minute).
6. Ensure the high pressure relief valve is functioning. (The circuit should develop a leak when the pressure is sustained above 75 cm H2O. By occluding the end of the circuit and squeezing the reservoir bag, a pressure of greater than 75 cm H2O can be created. When this is done, the high pressure release valve will open preventing any further increase in pressure in the circuit).
7. Unidirectional valves are functioning. (Watch the valves open and close smoothly as you take a test breath through the mask and anaesthetic circuit)
8. Check that the soda lime is fresh and that the canister is full.

D. Vacuum system:
Suction is connected and working.

E. Scavenging System:
Correctly connected to patient circuit.

F. Ventilator functioning.
(Test the ventilator using the 2 Litre reservoir bag as a set of test lungs. Once the system has been filled with fresh gas, turn the ventilator on. With the fresh gas flows at < 1 L/min, the bellows should continue to refill as the ventilator cyles. The maximal accepted leak is 1 L/min).

"SAMMM"	Preanaesthetic Check List	
Suction	Tonsillar tip connected to suction tubing and suction functioning.	✓
Airway's	Laryngoscope, blades, ETT, syringe, stylet, oral and nasal airways, tape, mask and manual resuscitation bag.	✓
Machine	Wall-source DHSS medical gas pipelines connected, N2O & O2 cylinder and pipeline pressures OK, Machine turned on, flowmeters functioning, O2 flush functioning, N2O and O2 proportioning device functioning, Oxygen pipeline disconnect (*Ritchie*) whistle functioning.	✓
- Vaporizer	Full and turned off.	✓
- Circuit	Assembled, valves functioning, and circuit leak less than 1 L / min at 30 cm H20 pressure.	✓
- Ventilator	Disconnect alarm functioning, and test ventilation leak of less than 1 L / min.	✓
Monitors	Capnograph connected to circuit and functioning. ECG, BP cuff, oximeter, peripheral nerve stimulator, and temperature probe monitors available and working.	✓
Meds	Intravenous fluids and equipment for starting i.v. prepared. Emergency medications as per staff anaesthesiologist where appropriate, (eg. atropine, ephedrine, succinylcholine etc.).	✓

CHAPTER 6

Intubation and Anatomy of the Airway

The goal of assessing a patients airway** preoperatively is to attempt to identify potential problems with maintaining, protecting, and providing a patent airway during anaesthesia. The assessment is performed with the aid of a physical examination and a review of the patients history and anaesthetic records.

The '1-2-3' test** is used to assess several factors that may affect decisions concerning the patient's airway management. The first component of the test is used to identify any restricted mobility of the temporomandibular joint (TMJ). Ask the patient to sit up with their head in the neutral position and open their mouth as wide as possible. Note the mobility of the mandibular condyle at the TM joint. The condyle should

rotate forward freely such that the space created between the tragus of the ear and the mandibular condyle is approximately one fingerbreadth in width.

The opening aperture of the patient's mouth should admit at least 2 fingers between their teeth. Note any loose, capped, or missing teeth as well as any bridge work on the teeth. If the opening is less than 2 fingerbreadths, it will be difficult to insert the laryngoscope blade, let alone visualize the larynx.

With the patient's tongue maximally protruded, the structures visualized should include: the pharyngeal arches, uvula, soft palate, hard palate, tonsillar beds, and posterior pharyngeal wall. Technical difficulties with intubation should be anticipated when only the

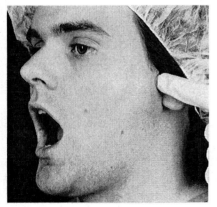

Fig.6.1: 1 = TMJ mobility.

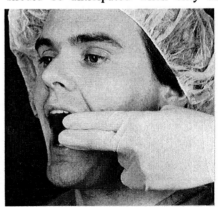

Fig. 6.2: 2 = Mouth opening.

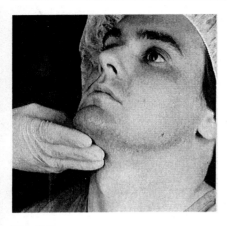

Fig.6.3:
3 = Thyromental distance.

tongue and soft palate are visualized in a patient during this above maneuver[1]. The third component of this test assesses the patient's thyromental distance. The thyromental distance is measured from the thyroid notch to the mentum (lower border of the chin).

Adults who have less than 3 fingerbreadths (or < 6.5 cm) between their mentum and thyroid notch may have either an anterior larynx or a small mandible, which will make intubation difficult.

Next, evaluate the mobility of the cervical spine. This is performed by asking the patient to flex and extend their neck. They should be able to perform this without discomfort. Disease of the C-spine (RA, OA, previous injury or surgical fusion) may limit neck extension, which may create difficulties during attempts to intubate. This is certainly true if the atlanto-occipital joint is involved, as restriction of this joints mobility may impair one's ability to visualize the larynx.

With the patient sitting upright with their head in the neutral position, mouth opened as wide as possible, and the

Samsoon's[3] classification of the visability of hypopharyngeal structures.				
	Class I	Class II	Class III	Class IV
Full view of the Uvula.	✔			
Body of Uvula visualized.	✔	✔		
Base of Uvula visualized.	✔	✔	✔	
Tonsillar Pillars	✔	(partial view)		
Tonsills	✔	(partial view)		
Posterior pharyngeal wall.	✔	✔	✔	
Soft palate and tongue.	✔	✔	✔	✔

Table 6.1: Hypopharyngeal Classification used In predicting a difficult Intubation.

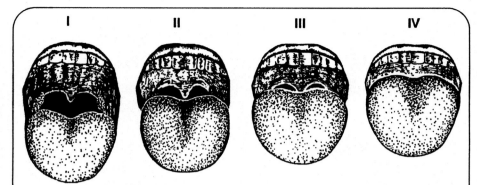

Figure 6.4:   Classification of the hypopharynx on the basis of the visible anatomy.   Class I - IV[2].

tongue maximally protruded, the airway can be classified according to the structures visualized in the hypopharynx[2] (figure 6.4, table 6.1).   In those patients who have a class I hypopharyngeal view, adequate exposure of the glottis during direct laryngoscopy should be easily achieved.   As the hypopharyngeal class number increases, so does the difficulty one anticipates in performing intubation using direct laryngoscopy. We can predict that a patient with a class IV hypopharynx, a full set of teeth, a restricted thyromental distance and restricted atlanto-occipital extension will be difficult to intubate using direct laryngoscopy.   Patients who have a restricted airway may require techniques other than direct laryngoscopy to secure an airway.   Choosing regional or local anaesthesia, rather than general anaesthesia, is one way to avoid the need for intubation.   Other airway management options include "awake" intubation with topical anaesthesia and intravenous

conscious sedation, or the use of a laryngeal mask rather than an endotracheal tube.

Finally one should try to ascertain whether there could be any difficulty with the lower airway (glottis, larynx, and trachea).   This is particularly important in patients who have had a previous airway injury, or surgery on their airway such as a tracheostomy. Observe the patient for hoarseness, stridor, or a previous tracheostomy scar suggesting a potential underlying tracheal stenosis.

Figure 6.5 illustrates the visualization of the laryngeal structures at the time of laryngoscopy.   Just as the visualization of the hypopharyngeal structures has been classified, the extent to which laryngeal structures may be visualized has also been graded from I to IV. While there is not a perfect correlation between the hypopharyngeal class and

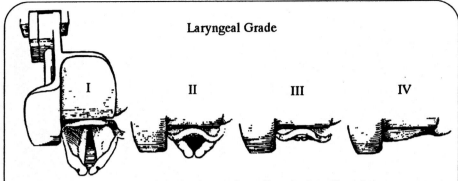

Figure 6.5: Laryngeal visualization and grading during direct laryngoscopy. (Grades I - IV). Adapted with permission from Cormack R.S., Lehane J. Anesthesia 39:1105 - 11, 1984.

the laryngeal grade, we anticipate that a patient with a class one hypopharyngeal view and no other identified airway abnormalities will have a grade I laryngeal view. Similarly a class IV hypopharyngeal view is a predictor of difficulty visualizing laryngeal anatomy.

The technique of tracheal intubation involves five steps**.

I. Positioning the patient.
II. Opening the patients mouth.
III. Performing laryngoscopy.
IV. Insertion of the ETT through the vocal cords and removing the laryngoscope.
V. Confirmation of correct placement, and securing the ETT tube.

I.   Positioning the patient
When preparing to intubate a patient, their head and neck should be positioned using a combination of both cervical flexion and atlanto-occipital

(AO) extension. We describe this as the *sniffing position*. This enables one to align the axes of the patient's mouth, pharynx, and larynx permitting direct visualization of the larynx during laryngoscopy (figures 6.6, 6.7, 6.8).

Atlanto-occipital extension alone increases the angle between the axes of the pharynx and the larynx. By con-

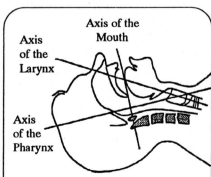

Figure 6.6: Poor alignment of the axes of the mouth, pharynx, and larynx in the neutral position.

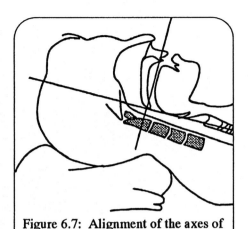

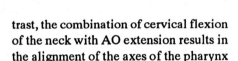

Figure 6.7: Alignment of the axes of the pharynx and larynx produced with cervical flexion.

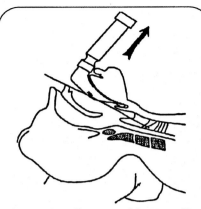

Figure 6.8: Alignment of the axes of the airway with cervical flexion and AO extension, permitting visualization of the larynx with direct laryngoscopy.

trast, the combination of cervical flexion of the neck with AO extension results in the alignment of the axes of the pharynx and larynx.

Optimizing the position of the patients head and neck before attempting laryngoscopy is an important initial step

in ensuring a successful intubation (figures 6.9, 6.10). This is especially true in obese or pregnant patients, or those patients in whom you anticipate a difficult intubation. It is good practice to make sure that your first attempt at intubation is your best.

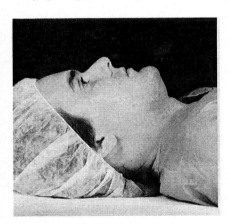

Fig. 6.9: Inadequate (supine) positioning for intubation.

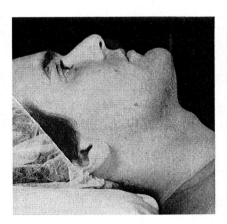

Fig. 6.10: Optimized positioning for intubation with cervical flexion.

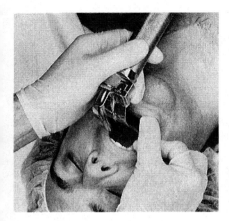

Fig. 6.11: Scissors technique.

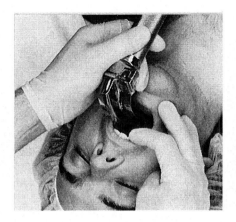

Fig. 6.12: Modified scissors technique.

Repeat attempts at intubation should be avoided unless there is something that can be done differently to improve one's chance of success. Persistent repeat attempts at intubation traumatize the patients airway, interrupt and delay both oxygenation and ventilation, and place the patient at risk of significant morbidity and mortality.

If you are having difficulty, retreat, regroup, and resume manual mask ventilation and oxygenation. Call for help and allow the patient to recover from any sedative - relaxant medications that have been given. No more than three attempts should be made at intubation. Discuss with your staff anaesthetist what other options are available for patients whom you anticipate will be difficult to intubate, or the patient in whom attempts at intubation have failed.

II.   Opening the patient's mouth
The next step in performing intubation is to open the mouth. Take the laryngoscope in your *left* hand as you stand directly behind the patient's head. The *right* hand is used to open the patient's mouth and, later, to advance the ETT. Mouth opening can be accomplished by using the *right* hand to open the patients teeth (e.g., the *scissors* technique, as illustrated in figures 6.11 and 6.12), or by placing the operators *right* hand on the patient's occiput to rotate the occiput backward and create AO extension (see figures 6.13 and 6.14). Using the *scissors maneuver* the index finger pulls the upper right incisors towards the operator, and serves to open the mouth, extend the atlanto-occipital (AO) joint, and protect the teeth and lips. At the same time, the thumb depresses the lower mandible, further opening the mouth. One can modify this technique by opening the patient's

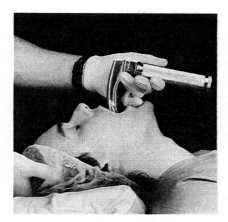 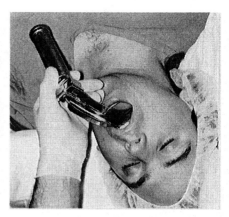

Fig. 6.13 and 6.14: Right hand controlling atlanto-occipital extension and facilitating mouth opening prior to laryngoscopy.

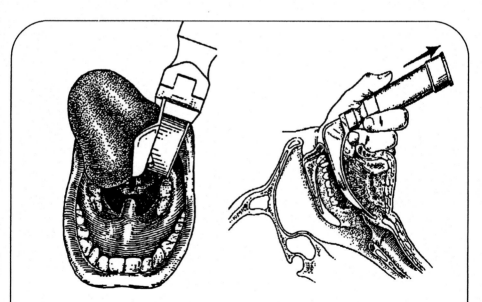

Figure 6.15: Illustrates the position of the curved laryngoscope blade, which displaces the tongue to the left. Upward and forward traction brings the larynx into view. Adapted with permission from Finucane B.T., Santora A.H. In: Principles of Airway Management. F.A. Davis Co., Philadelphia 1988.

mouth using one's right middle finger to depress the lower teeth (figure 6.12). If the clinician chooses the extraoral technique of mouth opening, their right hand is placed on the patient's occiput and the patient's head is rotated into the sniffing position. With this movement, the mandible drops and the mouth opens. This method of mouth opening is more suitable for the edentulous patient than the scissors technique.

III: Laryngoscopy

The third step involves insertion of the laryngoscope into the mouth (figure 6.15). The tip of the laryngoscope blade is advanced to the base of the tongue by rotating its tip around the tongue (figure 6.17). The laryngoscope blade should follow the natural curve of the oropharynx and tongue. The blade should be inserted to the right of the tongue's midline, so that the tongue moves toward the left and out of the line of vision. Avoid pushing the tongue into the back of the oropharynx, as this will also obscure your vision. Once the tip of the blade lies at the base of the tongue (just above the epiglottis), apply firm, steady upward and forward traction to the laryngoscope. The direction of force should be at 45^0 from the horizontal. Once the laryngoscope is properly positioned at the base of the tongue, avoid rotating it, as this action might exert pressure on the upper teeth and damage them. Damage to the immobile upper maxillary teeth is more common than to the lower mandibular teeth, which are free to move forward with the jaw during laryngoscopy. Figures 6.15 and 6.17 illustrate how the larynx is more visible if the blade of the laryngoscope moves the tongue to the left of the mouth and out of the line of vision.

Students learning the technique of laryngoscopy have a common tendency to adopt a stooped posture, which posi-

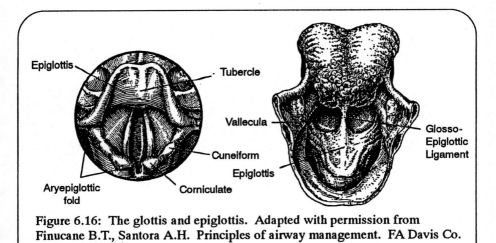

Figure 6.16: The glottis and epiglottis. Adapted with permission from Finucane B.T., Santora A.H. Principles of airway management. FA Davis Co. Philadelphia 1988.

tions their face within inches of the patient's. This posture limits the power that can be used by the arms, making laryngoscopy technically more difficult to perform. Try to maintain a good posture during laryngoscopy. This allows the arms to exert traction on the laryngoscope, rather than attempting to lift the laryngoscope with the wrists.

The larynx is located at the level of the 4th to 6th cervical vertebrae in adults. It consists of numerous muscles, cartilages and ligaments. The large thyroid cartilage shields the larynx and articulates inferiorly with the cricoid cartilage. Two pyramidal shaped arytenoid cartilages sit on the upper lateral borders of the cricoid cartilage. The aryepiglottic fold is a mucosal fold running from the epiglottis posteriorly to the arytenoid cartilages. The cuneiform cartilages appear as small flakes within the margin of the aryepiglottic folds (fig. 6.16).

The adult epiglottis resembles the shape of a leaf, and functions like a trap door for the glottis. In figure 6.16, the 'trap door' is shown in both its open and closed positions. The epiglottis is attached to the back of the thyroid cartilage by the thyroepiglottic ligament and to the base of the tongue by the glosso-epiglottic ligament. The covering membrane is termed the glossoepiglottic fold, and the valleys on either side of this fold are called valleculae. The valleculae are a common site for the impaction of sharp swallowed objects, such as fish bones. When performing laryngoscopy, one should advance the tip of the curved laryngoscope's blade to the base of the tongue at it's union with the epiglottis. Try to visualize this anatomy as well as possible when you perform laryngoscopy.

IV: Insertion of the ETT

Intubation is performed with the *left* hand controlling the laryngoscope blade, while the *right* hand opens the mouth and then passes the ETT tip through the laryngeal inlet. When a limited laryngeal view is encountered (grade III - IV larynx), the epiglottis can be used as a landmark for guiding the ETT through the hidden vocal cords. The tip of the ETT is passed underneath the epiglottis and anterior to the esophageal inlet. Recall that the glottis lies anterior to the esophagus (or above the esophagus during laryngoscopy). When the epiglottis partially obscures the view of the glottis, an assistant may be used to apply cricoid pressure. This maneuver moves the larynx posteriorly and helps to bring the vocal cords into view. A malleable stylet, shaped so that it forms a distal anterior *J* curve, can also be helpful in guiding the ETT tip through the laryngeal inlet. When you have had a limited view of the ETT passing through the vocal cords, the *Ford Maneuver* can help you to visually confirm its correct placement in the glottis. One performs this maneuver by displacing the glottis posteriorly using downward pressure on the ETT prior to withdrawing the laryngoscope. This maneuver is useful in the patient with a grade III or IV larynx for whom difficulty was encountered visualizing the glottic structures.

The cuff of the ETT should be observed passing through the vocal cords and

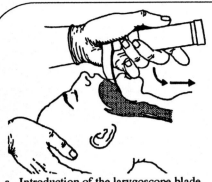

a. Introduction of the larygoscope blade using left wrist rotation.

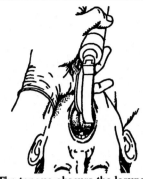

b. The tongue obscurs the laryngeal view due to inadequate advancement of the larygoscope blade .

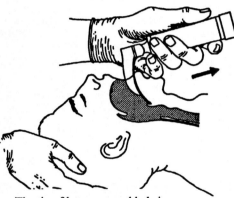

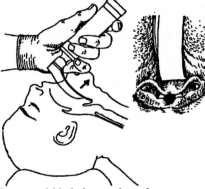

c. The tip of larygoscope blade is properly positioned at the base of tongue. The blade is lifted forward at 45 degrees.

d. Laryngeal blade inserted too deep, pushing epiglottis over laryngeal inlet.

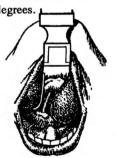

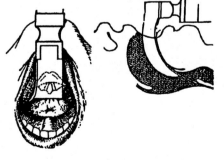

e. Laryngeal blade inserted to the left of midline, with tongue obscuring visualization of the larynx.

f. Laryngoscope blade inserted too far, with visualization of the esophageal inlet.

Figure 6.17: Laryngoscopy. Adapted with permission from Lui PL. Principles and Procedures in Anesthesiology. J.B. Lippincott Co. 1992

should lie just inferior (2 to 3 cm) to the cords. As soon as you withdraw the laryngoscope blade from the mouth, note the length of the ETT at the lips using the centimetre markers on the ETT. This may prove to be useful if the endotracheal tube moves from its original position. The usual distance from the tip of the ETT to the mouth is approximately 21 to 24 cm in adult males, and 18 to 22 cm in adult females. The usual distance for a nasally intubated adult male (from the tip of the ETT to the naris) is 25 cm. The ETT cuff is inflated with enough air to create a seal around the ETT during positive pressure ventilation. A cuff leak may be detected by listening at the patient's mouth, or over their larynx.

V: Confirmation of correct ETT placement.

Immediate absolute proof that the ETT is in the tracheal lumen may be obtained by observing the ETT passing through the vocal cords, observing carbon dioxide ($ETCO_2$) returning with each respiration, or by visualizing the tracheal lumen through the ETT using a fiberoptic scope. *Indirect confirmation* that the trachea is intubated with a tracheal tube includes: listening over the epigastrium for the absence of breath sounds with ventilation, observing the chest to rise and fall with positive pressure ventilation, and listening to the apex of each lung field for breath sounds with ventilation.   There are, however, numerous reports of physicians auscultating "distant breath sounds" in each lung field, when the ETT was, in fact, incorrectly placed in the esophagus. Hence, listening to the

lung fields may reveal bronchospasm or evidence of an endobronchial intubation, but cannot be relied on as absolute proof that the tube is correctly positioned in the trachea.

If the tube is positioned in the tracheal lumen and the patient is breathing spontaneously, the reservoir bag will fill and empty with respiration. If the patient is awake they will not be able to vocalize with an ETT positioned in the tracheal lumen. On an 'A-P' CXR the tip of the ETT should be located between the midpoint of the thoracic inlet and the carina.

Decreased air entry to one lung field may indicate that the ETT is in a mainstem bronchus (usually the right mainstem bronchus).   In this situation, the patient may become increasingly hypoxic, or continue to cough.   You may suspect an endobronchial intubation when you observe one side of the chest moving more than the other with ventilation.   In this situation, the airway pressures will be higher than normal (greater than 25 cm H2O), and an abnormally distant tube position at the patient's lips will be noted.

"IF IN DOUBT TAKE IT OUT:"**
This is prudent advice for anyone who has just intubated a patient and is unsure and unable to confirm the tube's placement. It is better to be safe by removing the ETT, resuming mask ventilation with 100% oxygen, stabilizing the patient, and calling for help, than to risk hypoxic injury and gastric aspiration.

"IF IN DOUBT LEAVE IT IN:"**

This advice applies to the clinician who is considering extubating a patient who has been intubated for a period of time. When the clinician has concerns as to whether the patient can be safely extubated (see chapter 7: extubation criteria), it is generally safer to delay extubation, continue to support ventilation, ensuring hemodynamic stability, analgesia, and oxygenation, than to prematurely extubate the patient.

Upper airway obstruction**:

The most common cause of an upper airway obstruction in an unconscious supine patient is from the tongue falling back into the hypopharynx (figures 6.18 and 6.19). In the unconscious state there is a decrease in the tone of muscles attaching the tongue to the mandible, hyoid bone and epiglottis. The respiratory efforts of the unconscious patient tend to pull the tongue backward causing further airway obstruction. Finally in the unconscious patient the epiglottis tends to fall downward, also increasing upper airway obstruction.

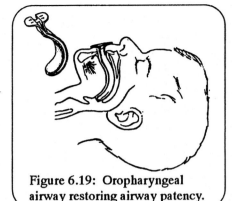

Figure 6.19: Oropharyngeal airway restoring airway patency.

Excluding intubation, simple maneuvers** to overcome upper airway obstruction in the unconscious supine patient, include:

1. Clearing the airway of any foreign material.
2. Using a chin lift maneuver.
3. Using a jaw thrust maneuver.
4 Inserting an oral and/or nasal airway.
5. Positioning the patient on their side in the semi-prone recovery position.

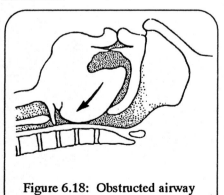

Figure 6.18: Obstructed airway in the unconscious supine patient.

References:

1. Mallampati SR, Gatt SP, Gugino LD, et al: A clinical sign to predict difficult tracheal intubation: A prospective study. Can J Anaesth 32:429,1985.

2. Samsoon GLT, Young JRB: Difficult tracheal intubation: A retrospective study. Anaesthesia 42:487,1987.

CHAPTER 7

Intubation Decisions

In chapter 6, we reviewed the technical skills required for tracheal intubation in adults. In this chapter we present four clinical cases as an illustration of the process used when deciding to intubate.

A clinician will readily recognize that the comatose patient with a severe head injury will need tracheal intubation for airway protection, maintenance, and hyperventilation. However, the need to intubate a dyspneic patient with chronic obstructive lung disease and a recent respiratory infection is not so readily apparent. Tables 7.1 and 7.2 list common criteria anaesthesiologists use to evaluate a patient's need for intubation. The individual criteria are not absolute indications. They are to be used together, in the context of the patient's clinical presentation, in formulating a decision concerning the patients need for intubation.

Case Studies on intubation decisions:

Case 1:
On the first day of your rotation, you are scheduled to assist with anaesthesia in the general surgical room. The first patient is a moderately obese forty year old female who is scheduled for an open cholecystectomy. What kind of anaesthesia should we provide for this patient? You ponder whether you should prepare equipment and medications for tracheal intubation.

Most open cholecystectomies today are performed under general anaesthesia with tracheal intubation. While it may be possible to provide regional anaesthesia (e.g., epidural anaesthesia) for this procedure most anaesthetists today will opt to provide general anaesthesia. The rationale for this decision includes:

1. A high abdominal incision with the need for muscle relaxation.
2. Surgical retractors which may impair spontaneous ventilation.
3. A moderately obese patient who will have difficulty breathing spontaneously when lying supine, due to the surgical retractors restricting the muscles of respiration.
4. Epidural anaesthesia used by itself would require a high level of block to provide adequate anaesthesia. This could impair the patients intercostal and abdominal muscles of respiration, resulting in respiratory insufficiency.

In the early days of anaesthesia, ether or chloroform was administered through a face mask during spontaneous respiration for this procedure. Ether produced marked muscle relaxation when used with minimal doses of muscle relaxants

Table 7.1 Objective Criteria for Intubation with or without ventilation* (Oxygenation / Ventilation / Mechanics)	
I. Oxygenation	• **PaO2 < 70 mm Hg** with FiO2 = 70% (A double flow puritan oxygen setup with 15 L/min x 2, provides a total of 30 L/min of oxygen flow to the patient, minimizing entrainment of room air; see figure 23.3, table 23.2).
	• **A-a DO2 gradient > 350 mm Hg.** Recall the normal A-a DO2 gradient is ≤ 15 mm Hg, and increases up to 37 with increasing age (Nunn Applied Respiratory Physiology 3rd Edition p. 248) Use an arterial blood gas sample, and alveolar gas equation to calculate A-a DO2 gradient; where: $PAO2 = (P_{atm} - P_{H2O}) \times FiO2 - PaCO2/0.8$
II. Ventilation	• **RR > 35 / min** in adults (muscles fatigue, at these rates).
	• **PaCO2 > 60** in normal adults.
	• **PaCO2 > 45 in status asthmaticus**, and rising despite maximum medical management (must use other objective and subjective criteria as well)
	• Respiratory acidosis with **pH < 7.20 in COPD** patients.
III. Mechanics	• **VC < 15 mL / kg** (Normal vital capacity = 70 mL per kg or approximately 5 litres; a vital capacity of 15 mL / kg is needed to cough effectively and clear secretions).
	• **NIF > -25 cm H2O** (Normal negative inspiratory force (NIF) is approximately -80 to -100 cm H20).

(e.g., curare 6 mg). Respiratory depression was accepted. When the ether was discontinued the patient recovered their muscle strength and increased their ventilation to match metabolic needs. Pulse oximeters, end tidal carbon dioxide monitors, nerve stimulators, mechanical ventilators, and antagonists for muscle relaxants were not available to the anaesthetist during these early years. Today, by contrast, we routinely plan general anaesthesia with intubation, muscle relaxation, and controlled mechanical ventilation for patients undergoing an open cholecystectomy. This allows the anaesthetist to produce pro-

Table 7.2 Subjective Criteria for Intubation and (or) ventilation* **(Protect / Provide / Maintain / T.B.T.)**	
I.	Real or impending **airway obstruction**. (e.g., epiglottitis, thermal burns, mediastinal tumours, etc.).
II.	**Protection of the airway**. (e.g., decreased level of consciousness, drug overdose, etc.).
III.	**"Tracheal bronchial toilet."** For patients who are unable to clear their secretions, the ETT provides a direct access for suctioning secretions, (e.g., COPD patient with pneumonia.)
IV.	To provide **positive pressure ventilation** during general anaesthesia. Additional indications for intubation under general anaesthesia include: long procedure anticipated, difficult mask ventilation, operative site near patients airway, thoracic cavity opened, muscle relaxants required, and if the patient is in a difficult position to maintain mask anaesthesia.
V.	Clinical signs of **respiratory failure** and fatigue. (e.g., diaphoresis, tachypnea, tachycardia, accessory muscle use, pulsus paradoxus, cyanosis, etc.).
VI.	**Shock** not immediately reversed with medical treatment (i.e. not responding to medical management in the first 35 - 45 minutes). Normal respiratory muscles use approximately 2 - 5 % of the cardiac output, in shock states this may increase to up to 15 - 20 %, stealing from other organs in vital need of oxygen such as the heart and brain. Dogs subjected to septic shock conditions, die much earlier if they are allowed to breathe on their own, when compared to dogs who are intubated and ventilated.

found muscle relaxation during the procedure, protect the airway from aspiration of gastric contents, and provide good ventilation and oxygenation. The anaesthetist can also administer potent anaesthetic drugs, such as opioids and volatile anaesthetic agents (e.g., isoflurane) to minimize the stress of the surgical procedure. Accordingly, you should plan to assist by preparing the endotracheal tube, checking the anaesthesia machine, and preparing the anaesthetic medications.

Case 2:
Having recently completed your anaesthesia rotation, you are working in the emergency department, when a pale diaphoretic 50 year old man stumbles through the door and collapses in front

of the receptionist. The patient is quickly placed on a bed and taken to the resuscitation room. Unable to find a pulse, the emergency physician immediately applies chest paddles, identifies a chaotic rhythm on the monitor, and defibrillates at 200, then 300 and finally 360 joules, in rapid succession. Unfortunately, the patient fails to respond. You are at the head of the bed and have initiated manual ventilation with an Ambu bag and mask. Chest compressions are initiated, while a nurse attempts, unsuccessfully, to insert an intravenous catheter. Should you proceed to intubate the patient?

The emergency physician appreciates your help and asks you to proceed with tracheal intubation. After placing the ETT, you confirm its position, secure it, and continue with controlled ventilation. At your suggestion, 10 mls of 1:10,000 epinephrine is injected down the ETT and propelled to the lungs and central circulation with subsequent ventilation. The cardiac rhythm changes to a coarser form of ventricular fibrillation. Repeat defibrillation at 360 joules converts the man's rhythm to a sinus tachycardia with a systolic pressure of 110 mm Hg. Frequent ventricular premature beats (VPB's) are noted, and lidocaine 100 mg is given through the now secure intravenous. An infusion of lidocaine is started and arrangements are made for the patient's transfer to the CCU.

The resuscitation of this patient could have proceeded with mask ventilation and chest compressions. By choosing to intubate this patient, we were able to protected the patient's lungs from the risks of aspirating gastric contents. The ETT also provided a route for administrating epinephrine, which played an important role in this man's resuscitation.

Later, a classmate asks why you didn't give any medications to intubate the patient. You explain that patients with profound cardiovascular collapse requiring emergent intubation, do not need any anaesthetic medications such as thiopental or succinylcholine to perform tracheal intubation. In fact the administration of thiopental could have a detrimental result by further depressing his already compromised myocardium. If your colleague asks what other medications can be given through the ETT, tell him to remember the word 'NAVEL'. This stands for the drugs: Naloxone, Atropine, Ventolin, Epinephrine, and Lidocaine, all of which can be given through an ETT.

Case 3:

Later, another clinical clerk asks for your opinion regarding a 68 year old man with known COPD. He is evaluating this patient in the emergency room because he is feeling more short of breath than usual. Your colleague was ready to send him home on antibiotics but hesitated after seeing his arterial blood gases (ABGs). He is concerned that this man may need to be intubated because his $PaCO_2$ is so high. On room air his ABGs were pH = 7.34, $PaCO_2$ = 65, PaO_2 = 54, HCO_3 = 34. How would you assess and treat this patient.

The patients ABGs demonstrate hypoxemia and an acute on chronic respiratory acidosis with metabolic compensation. You review his old chart and note that his HCO_3 was 33 and his PaO_2 was 59 mm Hg at the time of discharge 4 months previously. This, you suggest, probably represents his optimal blood gas values. You complete your evaluation by examining the patient noting a RR = 22 per minute, HR = 90 bpm, BP = 160/85, and diffuse mild rhonchi throughout the chest with no significant (i.e. < 10 mm Hg) pulsus paradoxus. You also note that the patient is able to talk without stopping frequently to catch his breath, and that he is not vigorously using his accessory muscles of respiration. Reviewing his other lab tests you note a Hb = 170, WBC = 12,000, and an ECG which is unchanged from his former cardiogram. The CXR demonstrates hyperinflation with basal bullae, but gives no evidence of cardiac failure or pulmonary infection. The patient admits to having stopped his bronchodilators in the last week. After clinical and subjective improvement with salbutamol (ventolin®) and ipratropium bromide (atrovent®), the patient is discharged home with a prescription for his inhalers and a follow-up visit with his family practitioner.

Case 4

Four weeks later you are completing your emergency rotation when the patient in the case 3 returns. You are alarmed at his ill appearance. His wife accompanies him and relates that he 'caught a cold' a week ago and has been getting progressively worse. He has been unable to eat or sleep for the last day because of his shortness of breath.

When you examine him you find that his breathing is laboured at 28 breaths per minute with a prolonged expiratory phase and a surprisingly quiet chest. He is diaphoretic, clammy, and has difficulty catching his breath to talk. His vital signs reveal a HR of 130 bpm, BP = 180/100, with a pulsus paradoxus of 35 mm Hg, and maximal use of his accessory muscles. The emergency physician orders salbutamol with ipratropium bromide by nebulization. An intravenous is established, ABGs are drawn, ECG, oximetry, and BP monitoring is initiated, and a portable CXR is ordered. Your classmate thinks you better intubate him now. Do you agree?

As the ABGs and CXR return, the patient is noted to have become increasing drowsy, while little clinical improvement has occurred. The ABGs on face mask oxygen at 8L/min reveal pH = 7.10, PaO_2 = 66, $PaCO_2$ = 120, and a HCO_3 = 36. The emergency physician orally intubates the patient using topical aerosol lidocaine anaesthesia to the hypopharnyx and glottis, and initiates hyperventilation at 20/min in order to 'blow off' the carbon dioxide. The nurse reports that the patients systolic pressure is now 65 mm Hg, and his cardiac monitor is showing sinus tachycardia at 120/min with multiple ventricular premature beats (VPB's). Your classmate reviews the CXR and states that he believes the patient has a pneumothorax on the left side. How are you going to manage the patient?

Before rushing to insert a needle thoracotomy and chest tube for a possible tension pneumothorax, you review the patient's status. Although he has become unresponsive to verbal stimulation, his trachea is in the midline, and you are able to manually ventilate him without excessive airway pressures. The emergency physician orders 100 mg lidocaine i.v., and asks you to take over ventilation while he reviews the chest radiograph. A repeat CXR is ordered to verify the ETT position. A fluid bolus of 1000 mL of ringer's lactate increases the patient's blood pressure to 100 mm Hg systolic. The VPB's remain but are now unifocal and less frequent. A mechanical ventilator is set up to provide ventilation, with an inspired O_2 concentration of 50%, a tidal volume of 850 mL, an intermittent mandatory ventilatory (IMV) rate of 12, and 5 cm of positive end expiratory pressure (PEEP).

Arrangements are made to transfer the patient to the ICU. Review of the initial CXR shows the previous basilar bullae, but no evidence of a pneumothorax. The second CXR shows the ETT tip to be correctly positioned in the mid trachea.

Your classmate was correct about the patient requiring intubation. Clinical examination, and ABG analysis confirmed that the patient was indeed in acute respiratory failure. Analysis of the ABGs revealed a severe acute on chronic respiratory acidosis. Often we have no background information regarding the patient's usual $PaCO_2$ and HCO_3 levels. In patients with COPD who may retain carbon dioxide, we rely on the pH more than the CO_2 to guide our management (as in case 3). A primary

respiratory acidosis, with a pH of 7.20 or less, indicates that the patient is no longer able to compensate. His condition was likely precipitated by his recent chest infection superimposed on his former severe COPD. $PaCO_2$ levels of greater than 95 mm Hg become increasingly anesthetic, (MAC CO_2 = 245, see chapter 14 re: MAC definition). The decreased level of consciousness may be accounted for by the low blood pressure and the high arterial carbon dioxide tension.

This case illustrates several common problems. The patient presented in an extreme condition, following an illness which likely resulted in significant dehydration. Upon his arrival in the emergency department, his cardiorespiratory system was being maximally stressed. Following intubation, his blood pressure fell precipitously. Patients with cardiorespiratory decompensation who require urgent intubation will often demonstrate a fall in blood pressure following intubation. This occurs irrespective of whether sedative drugs are given prior to intubation. The fall in blood pressure may be due to:
1. The sedative drugs given.
2. The removal of endogenous catecholamines by treating the condition that caused the patient to decompensate (i.e., removing the work of breathing from patient).
3. Decreasing venous return to the heart due to positive pressure ventilation.
4. All of the above, plus the unmasking of a significant underlying hypovolemia or concurrent illness (e.g., myocardial infarction).

The occurrence of multiple ventricular premature beats may reflect an irritable myocardium secondary to hypercapnia, hypotension, and hypoxemia. Another explanation for the appearance of the VPB's may be the result of an acutely induced hypokalemia. Mechanical hyperventilation may result in a precipitous drop in the $PaCO_2$ level. The sudden lowering of $PaCO_2$ will rapidly increase the patients pH and shift K^+ into the cells, creating an acute extracellular hypokalemia. The differential diagnosis of this patient's acute hypotension, dysrhythmias, and abnormal CXR includes a tension pneumothorax. In this case, the emergency physician correctly interpreted the lucency on the CXR as chronic basilar bullae, and avoided the potential disastrous consequences of a needle thoracostomy and chest tube insertion in this patient (i.e., risk of a bronchopleural-cutaneous fistula).

In retrospect, this patient fulfilled several criteria for intubation (Tables 7.1 and 7.2). This emergency was best met by first supporting his ventilation. As this patient's condition is likely to require prolonged ventilatory support, this is most easily accomplished by endotracheal intubation.

Typical Endotracheal tube sizes*
Adult male   8.0, 8.5, and 9.0 mm
Adult female   7.0, 7.5, and 8.0 mm

ETT size calculation for children:
Size (mm) = age/4 + 4.

The presence of a soft distal cuff on the ETT is equivalent to having a 1/2 size larger ETT. Endotracheal tubes less than 6 mm do not have distal inflatable cuffs. This decreases the risk of post intubation swelling and stridor, as a result of trauma from the ETT.

Example: A 10 year old child would generally use a 6.0 mm cuffed ETT, uncuffed tubes are generally used for patients age 8 and less.
6 yr. old child = 5.5 or 6 uncuffed ETT
Term newborn = 3.5 ETT
Premature infant = 2.5 - 3.0 ETT

Potential Complications of Intubation*:
Direct injury can be caused by either the laryngoscope, or the ETT. The lips, tongue, pharynx, larynx and trachea are all susceptible to injury. Damage to the teeth may be caused by the laryngoscope, or by biting on the ETT or tonsillar suction tip. Damage to the teeth, though rare, is still the most frequent problem resulting in litigation against anaesthetists. Damaged teeth can fragment and may be aspirated by the patient.

The patient who experiences a sore throat following their operation (with tracheal intubation), may obtain some relief with throat lozenges. This discomfort rarely persists for more than 24 hours. Beware of the patient who recalls a severely sore throat on previous operations. They may have a restricted airway, and their larynx may have been traumatized because they were difficult to intubate. Inserting the ETT through the larynx can injure the vocal cords or even dislocate the arytenoid cartilages. Patients with arthropathies, such as rheumatoid arthritis, may have an arthritic involvement of the arytenoids, creating a 'functional laryngeal stenosis'. If symptomatic, they may note hoarseness or pain on speaking. Always consider these patients to be at an increased risk for vocal cord and arytenoid injury, use a smaller ETT, and take extra care during intubation.

If the ETT is too short it may result in accidental extubation. Excessive advancement of the ETT into the trachea may result in an endobronchial intubation. Prolonged ETT placement may lead to vocal cord granulomas or tracheal stenosis. Although a cuffed ETT will protect against gastric aspiration, they do bypass the bodies natural humidifying and warming mechanisms, and afford a potential conduit for pathogens to enter the lung.

Upon inserting the ETT, a patient is subjected to a significant sympathetic stress, which may precipitate tachycardia, dysrhythmias, and myocardial ischemia. Pediatric patients have a relatively higher parasympathetic tone than adults. Hence tracheal intubation of infants and children may result in a significant bradycardia. In both adult and paediatric patients, medications are commonly given prior to intubation in an attempt to minimize these reflexes.

The most serious complication of tracheal intubation is an unrecognized esophageal intubation. The resulting gastric distension with ventilation, subjects the patient to hypoxia, hypercarbia, impairment of chest excursion, and increases the chance of regurgitation and pulmonary aspiration.

Criteria for extubation*:

The criteria for extubation are generally the reverse of those for intubation. The patient should not require an ETT for airway provision, protection, maintenance or tracheobronchial toilet, and should meet criteria for adequate oxygenation, ventilation, and lung mechanics. The condition that initially required intubation should be corrected prior to extubation. The patient should be able to protect their airway, i.e., they must be awake with a gag and cough reflex. They should be hemodynamically stable, and their RR should be greater than 8/min, and less than 35/min. Respiratory muscles will fatigue with prolonged rates greater than 35 breaths per minute. Oxygenation should be adequate, which means a PaO_2 of at least 60 mm Hg on an inspired oxygen concentration of 50% or less. This should be at accompanied with evidence of adequate ventilation with a $PaCO_2$ of less than 50 mm Hg. Vital capacity should be greater than 15 mL/kg (~ 1 litre in a 70 kg patient), with a tidal volume of greater than 5 mL/kg and the negative inspiratory force (NIF) should be more negative than -25 cm H_2O. The vital capacity, tidal volume, and NIF can be measured at the bedside with simple spirometry equipment.

CHAPTER 8

The Laryngeal Mask Airway (LMA)

What is the difference between a LMA and a tracheal tube*?
The laryngeal mask airway is a specialized airway device made of wide bore PVC tubing, which incorporates a distal inflatable non-latex laryngeal cuff (figure 8.1). The LMA is inserted without special equipment, in the back of the patient's pharynx with the soft laryngeal cuff resting above the vocal cords at the junction of the larynx and esophagus. An endotracheal tube (ETT) generally requires a laryngoscope for its insertion into the trachea. Unlike a LMA, the ETT passes through the vocal cords with its tip positioned in the mid trachea.

A foreign body in the trachea, such as an endotracheal tube, evokes an intense reflex. This results in an increase in heart rate, blood pressure and a cough reflex. The anaesthetist routinely administers potent anaesthetic agents such as opioids and muscle relaxants to blunt or abolish this reflex. The tracheal "foreign body" reflex does not result from the insertion of a LMA because it does not enter the trachea. Therefore, the LMA can be positioned with minimal amounts of anaesthetic agents (e.g., propofol alone). Maintenance of anaesthesia can be easily achieved by spontaneous respiration of a mixture of anaesthetic gases such as nitrous oxide and

isoflurane because the internal diameter of the LMA is relatively large compared to an ETT.

Does the LMA protect the patient against gastric aspiration*?
No. Should gastroesophageal reflux occur, the LMA will not prevent gastric contents from entering the trachea. (see chapter 24: Unusual Anaesthetic Complications: Aspiration Pneumonitis, and chapter 9: Perioperative Aspiration Risk: The Rapid Sequence Induction).

Which patients would be suitable for general anaesthesia with a LMA?
Patients who have no identified risk factors for aspiration (see chapter 9), and who do not require intubation and controlled ventilation, are suitable candidates for the LMA. It may be difficult to obtain an adequate seal using a face mask in patients with no teeth or with a full beard. The LMA is particularly useful in these patients, providing a good seal and an unobstructed airway.

Which patients are not suitable for a LMA?
1. Patients with *risk factors for gastric aspiration.*
   The comatose patient in the emergency department with a presumed drug overdose and intermittent airway obstruction, would not be a

Table 8.1: Advantages and Disadvantages of a LMA and Endotracheal Tube.

ADVANTAGES*	
LMA	**ETT**
• Easy to insert. • "Frees up" anaesthetist's hands, when compared to a face mask alone. • Provides a better airway in the unconscious patient than a face mask alone. • Can often be positioned with minimal anaesthetic drugs (e.g., Propofol alone, i.e., no *"Foreign body in trachea reflex"*)	• Provides airway protection against gastric aspiration. • Allows for tracheal suctioning. • Allows positive pressure ventilation without increasing the risk of gastric distension and aspiration.

DISADVANTAGES*	
LMA	**ETT**
• Doesn't protect against gastric aspiration. • Positive pressure ventilation with airway pressures of > 20 cm H2O results in increasing gastric insufflation and risks pulmonary aspiration of gastric contents. • Laryngospasm can occur with the LMA in place. This may result in complete airway obstruction.	• Muscle relaxants are usually required for intubation. • Technically more difficult to insert and position compared to LMA. • Trauma and positioning complications e.g., endobronchial intubation. (see chapter 8). • *"Foreign body in trachea reflex"*: resulting in an undesired reflex sympathetic stimulation (see text). • Laryngospasm can occur when the ETT is removed.

good candidate for the LMA, as they are at high risk for gastric aspiration.

2. Patients with *oropharyngeal or retropharyngeal pathology*, or foreign bodies in the hypopharynx. Examples include peritonsillar abscess, Ludwig's angina, epiglottitis, and trauma to the mouth.

3. Patients with *limited mouth opening*. (e.g., wired jaw, TMJ disease)
4. Patients with a *cervical vertebrae* or laryngeal cartilage *fracture*.
5. Patients requiring *positive pressure ventilation* with airway pressures of greater than 20 cm H20 (e.g., patients with significant restrictive or obstructive airway disease, trendelenburg position, laparoscopy).

A. The mask tip is pushed upwards against the hard palate as it is advanced into the pharynx.

B. With the neck flexed and head extended, the mask is advanced along the posterior pharyngeal wall.

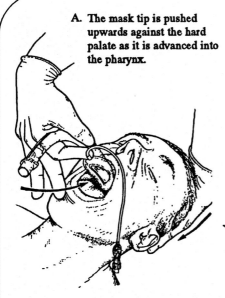 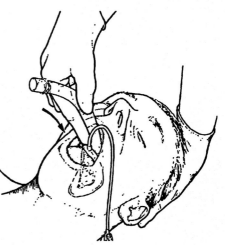

C. A correctly positioned LMA. The cuff should be inflated without holding on to the LMA.

D. When correctly positioned the LMA cuff does not push the epiglottis downward, or obstruct the glottis.

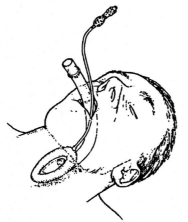 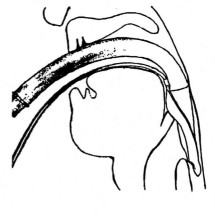

Figure 8.1: Positioning of the Laryngeal Mask Airway. Adapted with permission from Brain AIJ., The Intavent Laryngeal Mask Instruction ManuaL. Second Edition 1991.

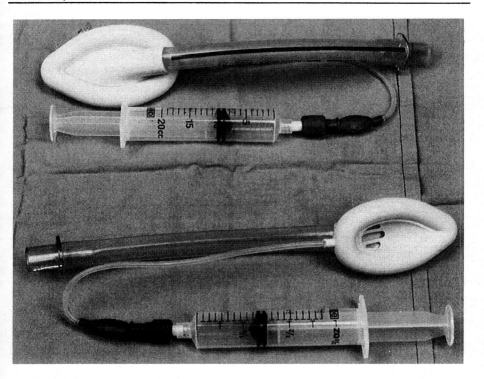

Figure 8.2: A number 4 (top) and number 3 (bottom) laryngeal mask airway.

How do you position a LMA?
The laryngeal mask is positioned after the induction of general anaesthesia. The laryngeal mask should be lubricated, and the cuff valve checked. It is recommended that the cuff is fully deflated prior to insertion. Our experience, however, has been that a small amount of air in the cuff (6 - 10 mL in an adult cuff) facilitates its insertion. The patient is placed in the supine position with their head and neck oriented in the usual 'sniffing position' used for intubation.

Anaesthesia is typically induced with the use of propofol. Other agents such as thiopental, ketamine or halothane can be used to induce anaesthesia. Propofol is the preferred induction agent as it is superior to thiopental for reducing laryngeal irritability and laryngospasm during LMA insertion. If thiopental is used for LMA insertion, the use of succinylcholine will facilitate its insertion and prevent laryngospasm.

After general anaesthesia is induced, the patient's mouth is opened by creating atlanto-occipital extension of the neck in combination with forward displacement of the jaw. The tip of the LMA is inserted into the mouth, and pressed up against the hard palate as it is advanced into the pharynx with the right hand. The cuff of the tube is guided along the posterior pharyngeal wall, and inserted as far as possible into the pharynx.

As an aid to advancing the laryngeal cuff past the tongue, it is recommended that the right index finger be positioned at the tube-cuff interface guiding the cuff into the pharynx, while the palm of the right hand pushes the proximal end of the LMA into the pharynx. Resistance is felt when the cuff is positioned at the upper esophageal sphincter. An assistant may help by holding the mouth open, or by lifting the jaw forward to open the hypopharyngeal space. The black line running longitudinally along the LMA tube should be facing the upper lip. Once in this position, the cuff is inflated with air, causing the LMA to rise out of the mouth a little as it settles into its correct position.

How do you remove the LMA?
The LMA can be left in place until the patient is awake enough to remove it. Alternatively the LMA can be removed by the anaesthetist as the patient is emerging from anaesthesia, or while they are under deep anaesthesia and breathing spontaneously. The cuff may be deflated before removing it. However, if left inflated, the cuff removes any upper airway secretions as it is taken out. Deflating the cuff risks having secretions stimulate the vocal cords with the potential for laryngospasm. Deflation of the LMA cuff in the lightly anaesthetized patient may result in laryngospasm because of stimulation of the vocal cords by secretions. Laryngospasm** is an involuntary reflex closure of the glottis by adduction of the vocal cords. It may result in the inability to

oxygenate or ventilate the patient, with secondary hypercarbia and hypoxemia. Stridor, a high pitched inspiratory sound produced by an upper airway obstruction, may be noted during laryngospasm. Occasionally a muscle relaxant, such as a small dose of succinylcholine, is needed to break the laryngospasm and permit positive pressure ventilation and oxygenation.

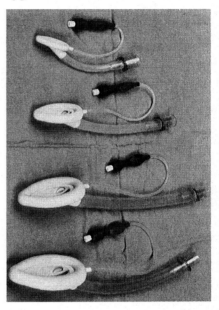

Figure 8.3: LMA Sizes and weights.
1: for wt. < 6.5 kg.
2: for wt. 6.5 - 25 kg.
3: for wt: 25 kg. up to adult females
4: for adult males

References:
1. Brain AIJ. The laryngeal mask - a new concept in airway management. Br J Anaesth 1983; 55:801-5.
2. Fischer JA, Ananthanarayan C, Edelist G. Role of the laryngeal mask in airway management. Can J Anaesth 39:1-3; 1992.

CHAPTER 9

Rapid Sequence Induction

A *'rapid sequence induction'** is used when a patient requires general anaesthesia who has been identified as having risk factors for gastric aspiration (see table 9.1). All patients are at risk of aspirating gastric contents when general anaesthesia is induced, because it impedes the patient's protective airway reflexes. For this reason, all patients requiring elective surgery are asked to abstain from eating solid foods for at least 8 hours, and clear liquids, for at least 4 hours prior to their procedure. Should gastric contents reflux into the hypopharynx during the general anaesthetic, the use of a cuffed endotracheal tube prevents it from entering the lungs.

The predisposing factors for gastric aspiration include a depressed level of consciousness ($\downarrow$LOC), impaired airway reflexes, abnormal anatomical factors, decreased gastroesophageal (GE) sphincter competence, increased intragastric pressure, and delayed gastric emptying. Patients who have any of these predisposing risks for gastric aspiration, and who require a general anaesthetic, should have measures taken to prevent aspiration during the perioperative period. The *three key components* of a rapid sequence induction are: preoxygenation, the application of cricoid pressure with loss of consciousness, and tracheal intubation with a cuffed ETT.

Without a cuffed tracheal tube, the patient is at risk of pulmonary aspiration of gastric contents. Cricoid pressure is applied by an assistant with the induction of anaesthesia. It's purpose is to reduce the risk of passive regurgitation and aspiration before an endotracheal tube can be placed. Cricoid pressure is only released when the tracheal tube cuff has been inflated, and the tube position confirmed by auscultation of both lung fields and measurement of carbon dioxide in the exhaled gases ($ETCO_2$).

Technique for Rapid Sequence*

1. *Prepare for General Anesthesia.* The suction is checked, on and under the patient's pillow. Airway equipment is checked. An appropriately sized ETT with a stylet is prepared. A laryngoscope and laryngoscope blade is checked. The machine is checked, the monitors applied, and the medications are prepared and labelled.

2. If a nasogastric tube is in place, suction and remove it, or leave it open to drainage.

3. *Preoxygenate* for 3 minutes with 100% oxygen or four vital capacity breaths with 100% oxygen.

4. The anesthesiologist may choose to administer a small dose of a non-depolarizing muscle relaxant (e.g., 1/10 intubating dose of rocuronium or ~ 5 mg per 70 kg) 3 minutes prior to induction to prevent excessive fasciculations from succinylcholine. This 'defasciculating' dose may be omitted in obstetrical patients, elderly patients, and pediatric patients.

5. A potent *opioid* may be given intravenously to blunt the sympathetic response to intubation (e.g., fentanyl, alfentanil, or sufentanil; the type of narcotic and its dose will vary depending on the patient's condition, procedure planned, and the individual anaesthetist's preferences).

6. A trained assistant, instructed in the correct application of *cricoid pressure,* should be positioned at the patients right side.

7. Anaesthesia for a *rapid sequence induction* is induced with a predetermined dose of a general anaesthetic agent followed by a muscle relaxant. This may be accomplished with a rapid injection of intravenous *thiopental (2 to 5 mg/kg),* or *propofol (1 - 2 mg/kg)* followed immediately with *succinylcholine (1.5 - 2 mg/kg).* Within 60 seconds of administration of succinylcholine, the patient will be anaesthetized, paralyzed, and ready for intubation.

With induction of anaesthesia the assistant applies cricoid pressure. Cricoid pressure is released when the positioning of the tracheal tube has been confirmed. In the event that the patient vomits during induction of anaesthesia, the assistant releases the cricoid pressure to avoid the possibility of esophageal rupture. The patient is placed in trendelenburg position, suctioned, and then intubated.

8. There are several options for maintaining anaesthesia once the patient is intubated. These include the administrating a volatile agent, N2O, opioids, sedatives, muscle relaxants, or intravenous general anaesthetic agents, such as propofol and ketamine.

9. If the plan is to extubate the patient at the conclusion of the procedure, precautions must be taken to prevent the possibility of aspiration during emergence from anaesthesia. The possibility of the patient vomiting and aspirating at the end of surgery is as great or greater than that during the induction of anaesthesia. To prevent this possibility, we attempt to have the patient positioned on their side, breathing spontaneously through the ETT, and responsive enough to open their mouth to commands to allow oral suctioning prior to removing the ETT.

Other anaesthetic agents may be used in place of thiopental to induce the anaesthetic state. These include ketamine 1 to 2 mg/kg iv, and propofol 1 to 2.5 mg/kg iv. Ask your staff anaesthetist

Table 9.1: Aspiration : Predisposing Factors and Preventative Measures**

↓ LOC	- Drug overdose (e.g., ETOH) - Anaesthesia	- Head injury - CNS Pathology - Trauma or shock states
Impaired Airway Reflexes	- Prolonged Tracheal intubation - Local anaesthesia to the airway	- Myopathies - CVA - ↓ LOC
Abnormal Anatomy	- Zenkers Diverticulum	- Esophageal stricture
↓ GE Competence	- NG tube - Elderly patient - Pregnancy	- Hiatus Hernia - Obesity - Curare
↑ Intragastric Pressure	- Pregnancy - Obesity - Bowel Obstruction	- Large abdominal tumours - Ascites
Delayed Gastric Emptying	- Narcotics - Anticholinergics - Fear, Pain, Labour - Trauma	- Pregnancy - Renal Failure - Diabetes
Prevention	- Preoperative Fasting - H2 Antagonists (↓ acidity) - Antacids (↓ acidity) - Metoclorpropamide (↑ motility) - Antiemetics - Regional or Local anaesthesia rather than General Anesthesia (GA)	- NG tube to empty stomach prior to induction - Cricoid Pressure on induction of general anaesthesia - Extubation awake on side

about the role of ketamine or propofol as alternatives to thiopental when anaesthesia is induced. Why is succinylcholine the most commonly used muscle relaxant for a rapid sequence induction? When would a muscle relaxant other than succinylcholine be chosen for a rapid sequence induction?

For a discussion of the consequences of pulmonary aspiration see chapter 24: Uncommon Anaesthetic Complications - Aspiration.

Notes:

CHAPTER 10

Monitoring in Anaesthesia

Inspection, palpation, percussion and auscultation are the cornerstones of monitoring in anaesthesia. In addition, numerous technical monitors are used to improve our understanding of the patients physiological status and minimize the patients anaesthetic risk.

ANAESTHETIC DEPTH*:

Patients undergoing surgery with local or regional anaesthesia are able to provide verbal feedback regarding their well being. When we induce a state of general anaesthesia, the onset of anaesthesia is signalled by the lack of response to verbal commands and the loss of a *'blink'* reflex when the eyelash is lightly touched. Inadequate anaesthesia may be signalled by facial grimacing to a painful stimulus or by movement of an arm or leg. In the case of full paralysis with muscle relaxants, inadequate anaesthesia is suggested by hypertension, tachycardia, tearing or sweating. Excessive anaesthetic depth may be signalled by cardiac depression manifesting as bradycardia and hypotension. In the patient who has not been given muscle relaxants and is breathing spontaneously, excessive anaesthetic depth may result in hypoventilation with hypercapnia (increasing $PaCO_2$) and hypoxemia.

Monitoring

Current Canadian guidelines to the Practice of Anaesthesia and patient monitoring are:

1. An anaesthetist present. "The only indispensable monitor is the presence at all times, of an appropriately trained and experienced physician."

2. A completed preanaesthetic checklist. (Current history and physical documented, appropriate laboratory investigations reviewed, pre-anaesthesia evaluation completed, ASA classification recorded, and npo policy observed if it is an elective procedure).

3. An anaesthetic record. Every patient receiving general anaesthesia, major regional anaesthesia, or monitored intravenous conscious sedation, should have their HR and BP measured at least every 5 minutes, unless impractical. The time, dose, and route of all drugs and fluids should be charted.

4. Oxygenation, ventilation, circulation, and temperature are continually evaluated both clinically and quantitatively. (Continual is defined as 'repeated regularly').

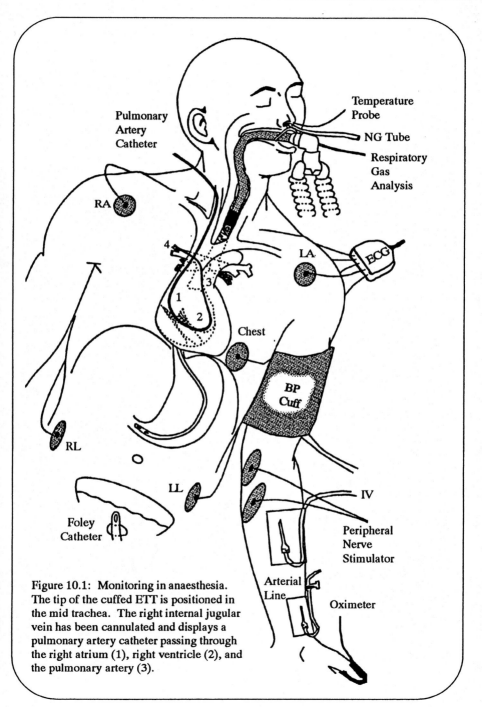

Figure 10.1: Monitoring in anaesthesia. The tip of the cuffed ETT is positioned in the mid trachea. The right internal jugular vein has been cannulated and displays a pulmonary artery catheter passing through the right atrium (1), right ventricle (2), and the pulmonary artery (3).

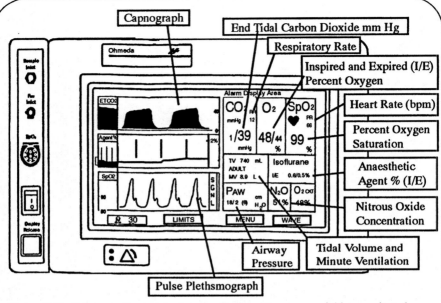

Figure 10.2: Intraoperative respiratory monitoring. Common variables monitored during general anaesthesia.

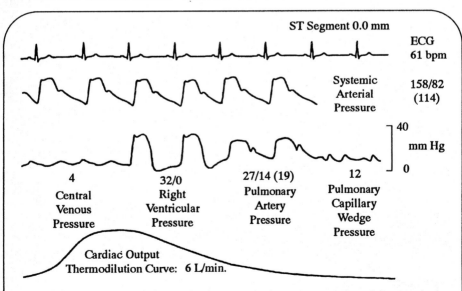

Figure 10.3: Hemodynamic monitoring. Central venous pressure, right ventricular pressure, pulmonary artery pressure, and pulmonary capillary wedge pressure tracings from positions 1, 2, 3 and 4 in figure 10.1.

I. OXYGENATION:

Oxygenation is monitored clinically by providing adequate illumination of the patient's colour and by pulse oximetry. The inspired oxygen concentration (FiO_2) is quantitatively monitored during all general anaesthetics using an oxygen analyzer. Each analyzer is equipped with an audible low oxygen concentration alarm.

II. VENTILATION:

Ventilation is monitored clinically by verification of a correctly positioned endotracheal tube as well as by observing chest excursions, reservoir bag displacement, and breath sounds over both lung fields. Ventilation is quantitatively monitored using end tidal carbon dioxide ($ETCO_2$) analysis as well as an audible disconnection alarm on all mechanically ventilated patients. The measurement of expired gas volumes and the ability to perform arterial blood gas analysis are useful adjuncts in assessing the adequacy of both oxygenation and ventilation.

III. CIRCULATION:

The circulation is monitored clinically by using one or more of: palpation of the pulse, auscultation of heart sounds, intra-arterial pressure monitoring, doppler pulse monitoring, or oximetry. Quantitative evaluation of the circulation includes an audible electrocardiogram (ECG) signal, and arterial blood pressure measurements at least every 5 minutes.

The ECG: A three or five lead electrode system is used for ECG monitoring in the operating room. A three lead system has electrodes positioned on the right arm, left arm, and chest position. Lead II is usually monitored with a three lead system, as the axis of this vector is similar to the P-wave axis. Identification of P waves in lead II and it's association with the QRS complex is useful in distinguishing a sinus rhythm from other rhythms. The chest electrode is usually placed in the left anterior axillary line at the fifth interspace and is referred to as the V5 precordial lead. A five lead electrode system adds a right leg and left leg electrode and allows monitoring of vectors I, II, III, AVR, AVL, AVF and V5 (see figure 10.1) Today's anaesthesia monitors are capable of analysis of the ST segment as an indicator of myocardial ischemia. Depression or elevation of the ST segment may be indicative of myocardial ischemia or infarction respectively. Over 85% of ischemic events occurring in the left ventricle during surgery can be detected by monitoring the ST segments of leads II and V5.

BP Measurement: The simplest method of blood pressure (BP) determination estimates the systolic blood pressure by palpating the return of the arterial pulse as an occluding BP cuff is deflated. Other methods include auscultation of the Kortokoff sounds with cuff deflation. This allows both systolic (SBP) and diastolic (DBP) pressure measurements. The mean arterial pressure (MAP) can be estimated from this as the MAP = DBP + 1/3(SBP - DBP).

Table 10.1: Normal values for a healthy adult undergoing general anaesthesia*.

Systolic Blood Pressure	SBP	85 - 160	mmHg
Diastolic Blood Pressure	DBP	50 - 95	mmHg
Heart Rate	HR	50 - 100	bpm
Respiratory Rate	RR	8 - 20	rpm
Oxygen saturation by pulse oximetry	SpO_2	95 - 100	%
End tidal carbon dioxide tension	$ETCO_2$	33 - 45	mmHg
Skin appearance		warm, dry	
Colour		pink	
Temperature		36 - 37.5	^{o}C
Urine production		≥ 0.5	$ml \cdot kg^{-1} \cdot min^{-1}$
Central Venous Pressure	CVP	1 - 10	mmHg
Pulmonary Artery Pressure	PAP (mean)	10 - 20	mmHg
Pulmonary Capillary Wedge Pressure	PCWP	5 - 15	mmHg
Mixed venous oxygen saturation	SvO2	75	%
Cardiac Output	CO	4.5 - 6	$l \cdot min^{-1}$.

Table 10.2: Derived Cardiopulmonary Values:

Body Surface Area (BSA)	Normal Values:
Mean Arterial Pressure	MAP = 80 - 120 mmHg
MAP = DBP + 1/3 Pulse pressure	
Cardiac Index (CI) = CO/BSA	$CI = 2.5 - 4.0 \ L \cdot min^{-1} \cdot m^{-2}$
Systemic Vascular Resistance	$SVR = 1200 - 1500 \ dynes\text{-}cm\text{-}sec^{-5}$
$SVR = \dfrac{MAP - CVP}{CO} \times 79.9$	
Pulmonary Vascular Resistance	$PVR = 100 - 300 \ dynes\text{-}cm\text{-}sec^{-5}$
$PVR = \dfrac{PAP(mean) - PCWP}{CO} \times 79.9$	
Stroke Volume $= \dfrac{CO \times 1000}{HR}$	$SV = 60 - 90 \ ml \cdot beat^{-1}$
Alveolar Oxygen Tension	$PAO_2 = 110$ mmHg ($FiO_2 = 0.21$)
$PAO_2 = (P_B - P_{H20})FiO_2 - PaCO_2/R.Q.$	(where $P_B = 760$, $P_{H20} = 47$, R.Q. = 0.8)
Alveolar-arterial oxygen gradient	A-aO_2 gradient < 10 mmHg ($FiO_2 = 0.21$)
$A\text{-}aO_2 = PAO_2 - PaO_2$	
Arterial Oxygen Content (CaO_2)	$CaO_2 = 21 \ ml \cdot 100ml^{-1}$
$= (SaO_2)(Hb \times 1.34) + PaO_2 \times 0.0031$	

Automated non-invasive BP measurements are routinely performed intraoperatively using a microprocessor-controlled oscillotonometer such as a Dinamap®. These units have replaced routine BP measurements by auscultation or palpation techniques. They automatically inflate the BP cuff to occlude the arterial pulse at preset time intervals. The cuff pressure is sensed by a pressure transducer. Repeated step deflations provide oscillation measurements which are digitalized and processed as the cuff is deflated. Rapid, accurate (± 9 mmHg) measurements of SBP, DBP, MAP and HR can be obtained several times a minute. Artifacts can occur with patient movement, arrhythmias, or blood pressure fluctuations due to respiration.

When automated non-invasive BP measurements are unsuccessful, simple auscultation or palpation techniques can be used with a manual cuff. Automated BP measurements are routinely performed every 3 to 5 minutes during general anaesthesia. Repeated rapid measurements for prolonged periods of time are not recommended due to a small risk of a compressive peripheral nerve injury.

Invasive monitoring of the circulation may include the use of an arterial, central venous, or pulmonary artery catheter. An arterial line is established with a small (20 - 22 gauge) catheter in a peripheral artery. The radial artery at the wrist is the most common site for an arterial catheter insertion. The femoral, brachial, and dorsalis pedis arteries are alternative sites for arterial line insertion.

Procedures frequently requiring direct *arterial pressure monitoring* include major cardiac, thoracic, vascular and neurosurgical procedures. Arterial line placement is also indicated in procedures requiring induced hypotension or induced hypothermia. Patients with co-existing diseases, including significant cardiopulmonary disease, severe metabolic abnormalities, morbid obesity, and major trauma, may also require perioperative arterial line placement.

A *central venous pressure* (CVP) catheter provides an estimate of the right atrial and right ventricular pressures. The CVP reflects the patients blood volume, venous tone, and right ventricular performance. Serial measurements are much more useful than a single value. The HR, BP, and CVP response to a volume infusion (100 - 500 ml of fluid) is a very useful test of right ventricular performance. CVP monitoring is useful in patients undergoing procedures associated with large fluid volume shifts. Shock states, massive trauma, significant cardiopulmonary disease or the need for vasoactive medications are other indications for using a CVP catheter.

Unlike a CVP catheter that lies in the superior vena cava, the *pulmonary artery catheter* (PAC) passes through the right atrium and right ventricle and rests in a branch of one of the pulmonary arteries (see figure 10.1). Inflation of a plastic cuff at the tip of the catheter allows occlusion of the proximal pulmonary artery and measurement of the distal pressure. This distal (back) pressure is referred to as the *pulmonary artery wedge pressure* (PCWP) and reflects the left atrial filling pressure. Thermodilution calculations of cardiac output are performed by injecting a fixed volume of cool fluid into the right atrial port and measuring the temperature change over time from a thermistor probe at the distal tip of the PA catheter. A sample of blood taken from the distal tip of the PA catheter can be analyzed to determine the mixed venous oxygen saturation (SvO_2). Detailed analysis of the patient's blood and fluid requirements, as well as the adequacy of oxygen transport can be made with the measurements obtained from a PA catheter. The results of manipulating the patient's hemodynamic parameters with ionotropic agents, vasopressors, vasodilators, diuretics, fluids or blood products, can then be followed.

Figures 10.2 and 10.3 illustrate typical cardiorespiratory variables monitored during general anaesthesia. Tables 10.1 lists normal cardiorespiratory values during general anaesthesia for a healthy adult. Table 10.2 lists formulas used in calculating common cardiorespiratory values.

IV. TEMPERATURE:

A temperature monitor must be readily available to continuously measure temperature. Temperature monitoring is mandatory if changes in temperature are anticipated or suspected.

An EKG with defibrillator, as well resuscitation and emergency drugs must be immediately available. In addition a peripheral nerve stimulator must be immediately available.

Cyanosis:

Cyanosis has been defined historically as the presence of 5 gm/dL of deoxygenated hemoglobin (deoxy Hb). When the hemoglobin level is 15 gm/dL and 5 gm/dL of this Hb releases oxygen to the tissues, the oxygenated hemoglobin portion (OxyHb) is 10 gm/dL. Hence the oxygen saturation is:

SaO_2 = OxyHb / (OxyHb + DeoxyHb)
SaO_2 = 10 / (10 + 5) = 66%

An oxygen saturation of 66% corresponds to an arterial oxygen tension of approximately 35 mmHg (see oxygen dissociation curve figure 10.4). Should the patient become anemic, however, the oxygen tension (PaO_2) at which cyanosis is detected will be even lower. Assume for example that the patient's Hb is now 10 gm/dL. The saturation at which we will detect cyanosis (i.e., when the DeoxyHb = 5 gm/dL) will be:

SaO_2 = OxyHb / (OxyHb + DeoxyHb)
SaO_2 = 5 / (5 + 5) = 50%

An oxygen saturation of 50% corresponds to an oxygen tension (PaO_2) of only 27 mmHg!

We now recognize that under optimal lighting conditions with no excessive skin pigmentation and a normal hemoglobin level, the earliest that cyanosis can be appreciated is at an oxygen saturation of approximately 85%. This corresponds to a PaO_2 of 55 mmHg. At a SaO_2 of 70% most clinicians will be able to detect cyanosis (PaO_2 of approximately 40 mmHg).

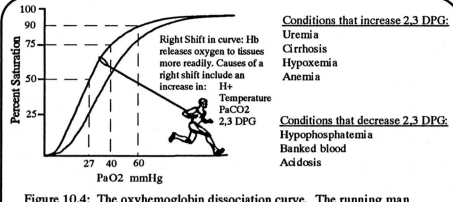

Figure 10.4: The oxyhemoglobin dissociation curve. The running man generates heat, carbon dioxide, and acid shifting the curve to the right, and enhancing oxygen release to his tissues.

Pulse Oximetry*:

Pulse oximetry allows beat to beat analysis of the patient's oxygenation status. Oximetry is based on the differences in light absorption by hemoglobin as it binds and releases oxygen. Red and infra-red light frequencies are transmitted through a translucent portion of tissue, such as the finger tip or earlobe. The signal is filtered to isolate pulsatile changes in light absorption. Microprocessors are then used to analyze the amount of light absorbed by the two wave lengths of light, and this is compared with an empiric table of measured values to determine the concentration of oxygenated and deoxygenated forms of hemoglobin. Once the concentrations of oxyHb and deoxyHb have been determined, the oxygen saturation can be calculated. Current pulse oximeters have numeric LED displays for the heart rate and percent saturation. A pulse plethysmograph allows visual analysis of the pulse waveform, while an audible tone, which varies with the percent saturation, allows an auditory assessment of the patients oxygenation status.

Pulse oximetry (SpO_2) includes measurements of oxyHb, deoxyHb, metHb, and carboxyHb. An over estimation of the true measured oxygen saturation (SaO_2) may occur in the presence of significant carbon monoxide poisoning (e.g., a burn victim). Oximeters may become inaccurate or unable to determine the oxygen saturation when the tissue perfusion is poor (e.g., shock states or cold extremities), when movement occurs, when dysrhythmias are present, or when there is electrical interference (e.g., electrosurgical cautery unit).

The oxyhemoglobin dissociation curve describes a sigmoidal shape (see figure 10.4). A decrease in PaO_2 of less than 60 mmHg (corresponding to a SpO_2 of

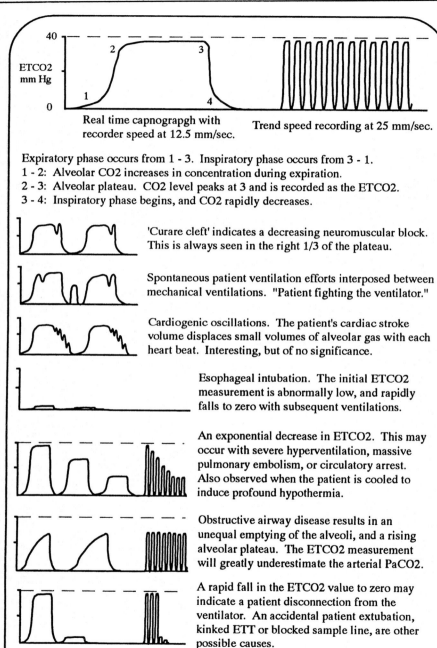

Real time capnograpgh with recorder speed at 12.5 mm/sec.

Trend speed recording at 25 mm/sec.

Expiratory phase occurs from 1 - 3. Inspiratory phase occurs from 3 - 1.
1 - 2: Alveolar CO2 increases in concentration during expiration.
2 - 3: Alveolar plateau. CO2 level peaks at 3 and is recorded as the ETCO2.
3 - 4: Inspiratory phase begins, and CO2 rapidly decreases.

'Curare cleft' indicates a decreasing neuromuscular block. This is always seen in the right 1/3 of the plateau.

Spontaneous patient ventilation efforts interposed between mechanical ventilations. "Patient fighting the ventilator."

Cardiogenic oscillations. The patient's cardiac stroke volume displaces small volumes of alveolar gas with each heart beat. Interesting, but of no significance.

Esophageal intubation. The initial ETCO2 measurement is abnormally low, and rapidly falls to zero with subsequent ventilations.

An exponential decrease in ETCO2. This may occur with severe hyperventilation, massive pulmonary embolism, or circulatory arrest. Also observed when the patient is cooled to induce profound hypothermia.

Obstructive airway disease results in an unequal emptying of the alveoli, and a rising alveolar plateau. The ETCO2 measurement will greatly underestimate the arterial PaCO2.

A rapid fall in the ETCO2 value to zero may indicate a patient disconnection from the ventilator. An accidental patient extubation, kinked ETT or blocked sample line, are other possible causes.

Figure 10.5: Capnography. A normal capnogram, and its four components are represented in the top figure. Examples of diagnostic capnograms are included.

90%) results in a rapid fall in the oxygen saturation. The lower limit of acceptable oxygen saturation is 90% as this represents an arterial oxygen tension just above hypoxic values.

End-Tidal CO_2 Monitoring
Definitions:
Capnometry: Is the measurement of the carbon dioxide (CO_2) concentration during inspiration and expiration.
Capnogram: Refers to the continuous display of the CO_2 concentration waveform sampled from the patient's airway during ventilation.
Capnography: Is the continuous monitoring of a patient's capnogram.

End-tidal CO_2 monitoring is standard for all patients undergoing general anaesthesia with mechanical ventilation. It is an important safety monitor and a valuable monitor of the patient's physiologic status. Examples of some of the useful information that capnography is able to provide include*:
1. Confirmation of tracheal intubation.
2. Recognition of an inadvertent esophageal intubation.
3. Recognition of an inadvertent extubation or disconnection.
4. Assessment of the adequacy of ventilation and an indirect estimate of $PaCO_2$.
5. Aids the diagnosis of a pulmonary embolism (e.g., air or clot).
6. Aids the recognition of a partial airway obstruction (e.g., kinked ETT).
7. Indirect measurement of airway reactivity (e.g., bronchospasm).
8. Assessment of the effect of cardiopulmonary resuscitation efforts.

Measurement of $ETCO_2$ involves sampling the patient's respiratory gases near the patients airway. A value is produced using either an infrared gas analysis, mass spectrometry, or raman scattering technique (see figure 10.2 and 10.5). Provided the inspired CO_2 value is near zero (no rebreathing of CO_2), the $ETCO_2$ value is a function of the CO_2 production, alveolar ventilation and pulmonary circulation.

During general anaesthesia the $PaCO_2$ to $ETCO_2$ gradient is typically about 5 mmHg. In the absence of significant ventilation perfusion abnormalities and gas sampling errors, an $ETCO_2$ value of 35 mmHg will correspond to a $PaCO_2$ value of approximately 40 mmHg. Increases or decreases in $ETCO_2$ values may be the result of either increased CO_2 production or decreased CO_2 elimination (see table 10.3).

Monitoring Neuromuscular function: In order to quantify the depth of neuromuscular blockade, electomyography is commonly employed during anaesthesia. This involves the application of two electrodes over an easily accessed peripheral nerve. The ulnar nerve is the most common nerve used for monitoring neuromuscular function during general anaesthesia. Other nerves that may be used include the facial nerve and the common peroneal nerve. The electrodes are attached to a nerve stimulator, which applies an electrical impulse to the nerve. By attaching a strain gauge to the muscle being stimulated, the muscle response to stimulation may be observed or measured. Ulnar nerve stimulation

Table 10.3: Etiologies of increased or decreased ETCO$_2$ values (Modified from Gilber HC, Vendor JS. Monitoring the Anesthetized Patient. In Clinical Anesthesia. Second Edition 1993. JB Lippincott Co. Philadelphia).

Increased ETCO$_2$	Decreased ETCO$_2$
Changes in CO$_2$ Production	
Hyperthermia Sepsis, Thyroid storm Malignant Hyperthermia Muscular Activity	Hypothermia Hypometabolism
Changes in CO$_2$ Elimination	
Hypoventilation Rebreathing	Hyperventilation Hypoperfusion Embolism

results in the contraction of the abductor pollicis muscle and a twitch in the thumb. Up to 70% of the neuromuscular receptors may be blocked by a neuromuscular blocking drug before a change in the twitch height can be observed. When 90% of the receptors are blocked, all observable twitches are eliminated.

Common methods of stimulation of the nerve include a single twitch stimulus, four twitch stimuli, (each separated by 1/2 second) referred to as a train-of-four stimulus (TOF), or a continuous stimulus referred to as a tetanus stimulation. The intensity of neuromuscular blockade and type of blockade (i.e., depolarizing versus a non-depolarizing blockade) can be characterized by the response to these different type of stimuli. Clinical relaxation will occur when a single twitch or first twitch of a TOF stimulus, is reduced by 75% to 95% of its original height (see figure 10.6).

A pure depolarizing block produces a uniform reduction in the height of a single twitch, TOF stimulus, and tetanus stimulation. If excessive amounts of succinylcholine are given (> 5-6 mg/kg), the block may begin to resemble a non-depolarizing block and is said to be a phase II block (see succinylcholine). Tetanus stimulation of a nerve will demonstrate a continued weak contraction in the presence of a depolarizing block, but will progressively fade with a non-depolarizing block.

In the case of a non-depolarizing blockade, there is an increasing reduction in each of the four TOF twitches. The ratio of height of the fourth to first twitch (i.e., the TOF ratio) is less than 0.7 in a non-depolarizing block. Also both the single twitch and the TOF stimulus, will be increased following a tetanus stimulation. This is referred to as post-tetanic facilitation, and only occurs with a non depolarizing block.

The intensity of non-depolarizing neuromuscular blockade can be estimated by the height and number of twitches that are present following a TOF stimulus. When the first twitch is reduced in height by 75%, the fourth twitch disappears. With an 80% reduction in height of the first twitch both the third and fourth twitches are lost, and with a 90% reduction in the first twitch the remaining three twitches disappear.

When all twitches disappear ≥ 90% of all receptors are occupied. For procedures requiring muscle relaxation attempts are made to maintain one twitch present with a TOF stimulus. Reversal of a neuromuscular block will be easily accomplished if all four twitches of the TOF are present, and will be difficult or impossible if one or no twitches are observed.

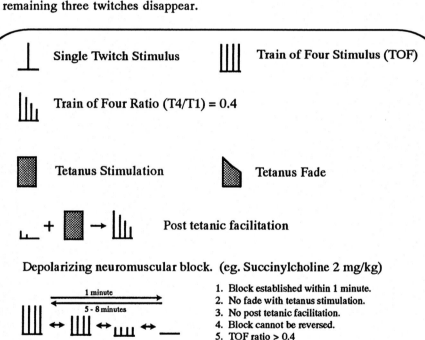

Figure 10.6 Assessing neuromuscular function. Characteristics of a depolarizing and non-depolarizing neuromuscular block.

Notes:

CHAPTER 11

Intravenous Anaesthetic Agents

For over forty years, the ultra short acting thiobarbiturate, sodium thiopental, has been the intravenous induction agent of choice. Thiopental's popularity is currently being challenged by a new akylphenol class of drug called propofol. Propofol's rapid metabolism and elimination, as well as its anti-emetic properties, are welcome features to the specialty of anaesthesia. Ketamine is infrequently used as an intravenous induction agent due to its unpopular psychological side effects. Despite this, it continues to play an important role in anaesthesia due to its unique cardiorespiratory pharmacodynamics.

In this chapter we shall present three commonly used intravenous anaesthetic induction agents: thiopental, propofol, and ketamine. For each of these drugs we shall highlight its physical properties, pharmacokinetics, pharmacodynamics, dosage, indications and contraindications. Other adjuvant intravenous anaesthetic agents such as midazolam and droperidol are also presented. Opioid analgesics and neuromuscular blocking agents are presented in the following chapters.

A. Sodium Thiopental (Pentothal®)
Definition:
Ultra short acting barbiturate

Classification:
Intravenous anaesthetic - hypnotic

Physical Chemical Properties:
Thiopental is a highly lipid soluble compound, that is supplied as a yellow powder with a sulphuric smell and a bitter taste. When combined with sodium carbonate, it becomes water soluble. It is bacteriostatic in water and has a pH of 10.6 to 10.8. When injected, sodium carbonate is neutralized and the thiopental is converted to its lipid soluble non ionized form (pKa = 7.6, i.e. 40% ionized at pH = 7.4). Thiopental is highly protein bound by albumen (75%), which prevents its precipitation out of solution in vivo.

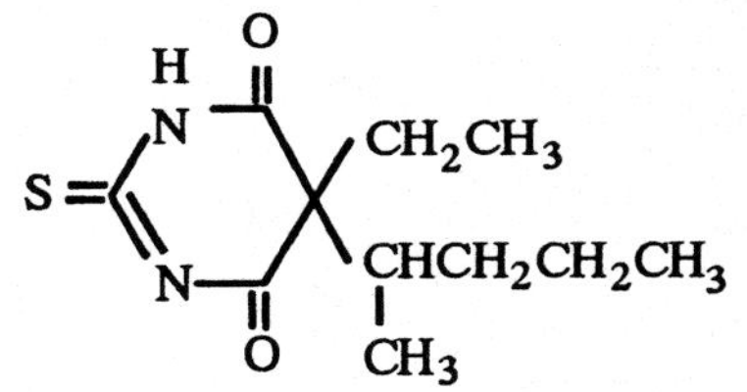

Figure 11.1: Sodium thiopentothal.

Supplied: Thiopental is supplied in the form of a yellow powder, dissolved in water and sodium carbonate to make a

2.5% solution (25 mg/ml). It is stable as a solution at room temperature for a period of 2 weeks.

Structure Activity Relationship:

· CH3 at N-1: shortens the duration
      (eg. methohexital)
· S substitution at C-2:
      markedly shortens the duration of narcosis
· C-5 substitution with branched chains:
      increases potency and toxicity

Pharmacokinetics: (i.e., What happens to the drug with respect to uptake, distribution, metabolism, and excretion.)

An intravenous dose of 3 - 5 mg/kg results in loss of consciousness. The time required to render the patient unconscious is generally 30 to 60 seconds following administration. This time has been referred to as the 'arm-brain' circulation time. It is the time required for the drug to pass from the site of injection to the brain as it passes through the right heart, pulmonary circulation, and left heart. When no other drugs are given, the anaesthetic state persists for 5 to 10 minutes. The patient awakes after this period of time not because the drug has been metabolized (T½ = 5 - 12 hours), but rather because the thiopental has moved away from the brain and is entering the more slowly perfused organs. Hence, the termination of action of the drug is due to its 'redistribution' from the brain to other tissues and organs.

The brain, liver, kidney's, and adrenal glands comprise the vessel rich group*. They receive 75% of the cardiac output, even though they constitute only 10% of body mass. After reaching its peak serum level within these vessel rich organs, thiopental is then distributed to the muscles, fat and the vessel poor group of organs (see figure 11.2). The muscle group receives just less than 20% of the cardiac output (second only to the vessel rich group), and constitutes approximately 50% of the body mass. While peak serum concentrations of thiopental are reached within seconds of the injection, the fat group and vessel poor group (e.g., bone, and cartilage) may require hours before peak levels are achieved. The longer time for thiopental to reach peak levels in these compartments is due to the lower perfusion rates of the vessel poor organs.

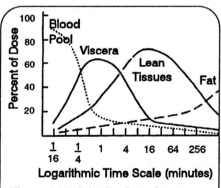

Figure 11.2 Distribution of thiopentothal in the vessel rich and vessel poor groups over time, following a rapid intravenous injection. (Modified with permission from Miller RD., Anesthesia 3rd Ed. Churchill Livingstone 1990).

Sulphur containing drugs, acidosis, and non steroidal anti-inflammatory drugs (NSAIDS) may displace thiopental from albumen. This results in an increase in free thiopental which increases the anaesthetic potency and toxicity. Liver and renal disease may be associated with lower albumen levels, also raising free serum thiopental concentrations.

Metabolism occurs primarily in the liver with approximately 10 to 15% of the remaining drug level being metabolized per hour. A desulfuration reaction occurring in the liver produces pentobarbital, which then undergoes oxidative metabolism yielding two compounds with no anaesthetic activity. Less than one per cent of the administered thiopental is excreted unchanged in the urine.

Pharmacodynamics: (i.e., What the drug does in the body.)

CNS:
Barbiturates, including thiopental, interact with chloride ion channels by altering the duration they spend in an 'open state'. This facilitates inhibitory neurotransmitters such as gama amino butyric acid (GABA), as well as blocking excitatory neurotransmitter actions such as glutamic acid.

Thiopental will decrease both cerebral electrical and metabolic activity. Hence, it can be used to stop seizure activity in an emergency situation. To maintain depression of cerebral electrical activity, very high doses of thiopental are required. To maintain seizure control and avoid significant

cardiovascular depression from high doses of thiopental, other antiepileptic drugs are used (e.g., a benzodiazepine class of drug).

Elevated intracranial pressure (ICP) can be quickly reduced by administering thiopental. The improvement in ICP is transitory and would require excessive amounts of thiopental to maintain. The use of high doses of barbiturates in patients with persistently elevated ICP, has not been shown to improve their overall outcome. The reduction of ICP from thiopental is a result of cerebral vasoconstriction, reduced cerebral metabolism and oxygen requirements. This is associated with a decrease in cerebral blood volume. The overall effect is an improvement in cerebral perfusion pressure (CPP), as the decrease in ICP is generally greater than the decrease in mean arterial pressure (MAP).

$$\uparrow CPP = \downarrow MAP - \downarrow\downarrow ICP$$

Thiopental has an anti-analgesic effect, since low doses may decrease a patients pain threshold.

Intraocular pressure (IOP) decreases up to 25% with 3 - 5 mg/kg of thiopental. The decrease in IOP persists for 3 to 5 minutes.

CVS:
Thiopental causes a dose related depression of myocardial function as measured by cardiac output (CO), stroke volume (SV), and blood pressure. Coronary blood flow, heart rate, and myocardial oxygen uptake all increase

following administration of thiopental. Venous tone decreases (decreased pre-load) and contributes to the increase in HR, and decrease in BP. Little change in the total peripheral resistance occurs following thiopental administration.

RESP:

Induction of anaesthesia with thiopental may be associated with 2 or 3 large breaths followed by apnea. The duration of apnea following a 'sleep' dose of thiopental is usually less than one minute. There is a dose related depression of the respiratory response to hypercarbia and hypoxia. Laryngospasm may occur with induction, especially at light levels of anaesthesia and with airway manipulation. Bronchoconstriction may be associated with thiopental, but is much more commonly seen following the combination of a small dose of thiopental with airway manipulation or intubation. As with any general anaesthetic agent, the functional residual capacity (FRC) is reduced with the induction of anaesthesia by up to 20%.

GI:

Enzyme induction may occur with prolonged high dose therapy, as in barbiturate induced comas. Hypoalbuminemia will result in an increase in unbound (free) thiopental and an increase in the potency of thiopental.

GU/Pregnancy/Fetus:

Thiopental has little or no effect on the kidney's or gravid uterus. Although thiopental rapidly crosses the placenta to reach the fetus, it has no significant effect on the fetus when used for cesarean section provided the dose used is limited to 4 mg/kg.

Dose and Administration:

Thiopental must be used with caution in patients suffering from a shock state. This was quickly appreciated by the anaesthetists caring for the casualties of pearl harbour. They presented to the operating room in shock states secondarily to massive blood loss. The administration of the usual sleep dose of thiopental of 3 to 6 mg/kg for induction of anaesthesia resulted in their rapid demise. For a frail elderly lady who has fractured her hip, a dose of 25 to 50 mg (0.5 - 1 mg/kg) may be all that is required for the induction of anaesthesia. For short procedures (eg. cardioversion) a dose of 2 mg/kg is generally sufficient.

Indications:

1. Sole anaesthetic agent for brief surgical procedures (less than 15 minutes).
2. For induction of anaesthesia, prior to administration of other anaesthetic agents.
3. For control of convulsive states.
4. For the supplementation of regional anaesthesia, or low potency anaesthetic agents such as N2O.

Contraindications to Thiopental*:

I. ABSOLUTE:

1. Lack of knowledge of the drug.
2. Lack of resuscitative equipment.
3. Inability to maintain a patent airway.
4. Complete absence of suitable veins.
5. Allergy or hypersensitivity to barbiturates.
6. Status asthmaticus.
7. Porphyria (Varigate Porphyria, or Acute Intermittent Porphyria)

II. RELATIVE:
1. Hypotension or shock.
2. Severe cardiovascular disease.
3. Severe liver disease.
4. Myxedema.

Side Effects and Toxicity:
An extravascular injection of thiopental will usually not cause any serious long term sequelae, provided the concentration of the solution injected is ≤ 2.5%. With more concentrated solutions, an extravascular injection may cause severe pain on injection as well as subsequent tissue necrosis. If a solution of ≥ 2.5% thiopental is injected accidentally into an artery, severe pain, vascular spasm, loss of digital pulses, gangrene, and permanent nerve damage may occur. If an intra-arterial injection does occur, the offending iv should be kept in place, and 5 to 10 mL of 1% plain lidocaine administered through it. Consideration should be given for systemic heparin administration (to prevent thrombosis), and for administering some form of sympathetic block (eg. stellate ganglion block) to reduce the sympathetic tone of the injured area.

Other side effects not mentioned above include allergic reactions, which may manifest as a skin rash, pain on injection, urticaria, angioedema, bronchospasm, laryngospasm, and cardiovascular collapse.

B. Propofol (Diprivan®)
Definition:
Intravenous anaesthetic - hypnotic
Classification: Akylphenol
Physical Chemical Properties:

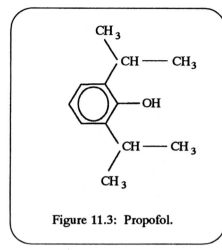

Figure 11.3: Propofol.

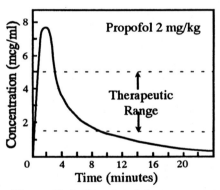

Figure 11.4: Simulated time course of whole-blood levels of propofol following an induction dose of 2.0 mg/kg. (With permission from Miller RD., Anesthesia 3rd Ed. Churchill Livingstone, 1990.)

    1% propofol (10 mg/mL)
    10% soyabean oil
    2.25% glycerol
    1.2% purified egg phosphatide

Propofol is a highly lipid soluble oil that is combined with glycerol, egg, and soyabean oil for intravenous administration. It's appearance is similar to that of 2% milk, as the solution that is used to dissolve it is similar to total parenteral nutrition (TPN) solutions. It has a pH of 7 and is supplied in 20 mL ampules with a concentration of 10 mg/ml.

Pharmacokinetics:
T½ initial distribution = 2 - 8 minutes.
T½ redistribution = 30 - 60 minutes.
T½ elimination = 4 - 7 hours.

Following a single bolus injection, peak serum concentrations are reached rapidly. Propofol's high lipid solubility results in a quick transfer to the brain and rapid onset (one 'arm-brain' circulation time). Recovery from a single bolus injection results from both redistribution and elimination. Propofol is metabolized in the liver, yielding water soluble inactive conjugated compounds which are excreted by the kidney. Less than 2% of propofol is excreted unchanged in the urine and feces. Propofol is cleared from the blood faster than hepatic blood flow, which suggests that extrahepatic metabolism and elimination may be occurring in the lungs.

Pharmacodynamics:

CNS:
Unlike barbiturates, propofol is not antanalgesic. At low (subhypnotic) concentrations, propofol can provide both sedation and amnesia. Patients report a general sense of well being on awakening from propofol anaesthesia. Intracranial and intraocular pressure are both decreased by propofol. Cerebral perfusion pressure undergoes a small decrease with propofol. The cerebral blood vessels remain responsive to CO2 during a propofol infusion. Cerebral metabolic rate is decreased up to 36%. Propofol appears to have neither epileptic nor anticonvulsant properties.

RESP:
The respiratory rate is decreased with the induction of anaesthesia, and approximately one quarter of patients become apneic at induction. The period of apnea depends on the dose given, the speed of injection, and concomitant use of an opioid. The frequency of apnea is greater than that seen following thiopental. Maintenance anaesthesia (100 mcg/kg/min iv) with propofol results in a decreased tidal volume and increased respiratory rate. At this same infusion rate the ventilatory response to CO2 is depressed similar to that caused by administration of 1 MAC (0.76%) halothane. Unlike halothane, however, doubling the infusion rate of propofol does not result in a marked increase in depression of the CO2 response curve.

CVS:
Systolic, mean and diastolic blood pressure are reduced 25-40% with an induction dose of 2-2.5 mg/kg. Cardiac output, stroke volume and systemic vascular resistance are all decreased with induction by 15-20%. The decrease in blood pressure is believed to be secondary to both myocardial depression and vasodilation. Heart rate may increase, remain the same, or decrease following propofol. Concomitant administration of an opioid tends to result in a greater reduction in heart rate, cardiac output, and arterial pressure.

OTHERS:
Propofol neither precipitates histamine release, nor triggers malignant hyperthermia. Propofol has no effect on muscle relaxants and is associated with a low incidence of nausea and vomiting. Pain on injection is more common than with thiopental, especially if given in a small vein in the hand. The discomfort at injection can be decreased by the administration of a small dose of lidocaine with propofol, or by administering propofol through a fast flowing more proximal intravenous catheter.

Intravenous Induction Dose:
An induction dose of 2.5 - 3.0 mg/kg is used for healthy unpremedicated patients. When an opioid, or a premedication has been given, the induction dose is reduced to 1.5-2.0 mg/kg. In elderly patients the induction dose should be reduced to ≤ 1 mg/kg of propofol.

Infusion rates of 50-150 mcg/kg/min in combination with nitrous oxide and opioids, can be used for maintenance of anaesthesia.

Intravenous conscious sedation for operative procedures with local anaesthesia can be facilitated with propofol infusions of 25 - 75 mcg/kg/min.

Contraindications to Propofol*:
1. Allergy (egg allergy).
2. Lack of resuscitation equipment or knowledge of the drug.
3. Inability to maintain a patent airway.
4. Conditions in which precipitous reductions in blood pressure would not be tolerated; in patients with a fixed cardiac output (severe aortic or mitral stenosis, IHSS, pericardial tamponade) and those in shock states.

C. Ketamine (Ketalar®)

Definition/Classification:
Dissociative Anaesthetic Agent

Physical Chemical Properties:
Ketamine is chemically related to the psychotropic drug phencyclidine (PCP), and cyclohexamine. It is water soluble and is 10 times more lipid soluble than thiopental. It exists as two enantiomers s (+) and r (-) ketamine, and is supplied as a 50:50 mixture. It has a pH of 3.5 - 5.5 and is supplied as a clear colourless solution of 10 and 50 mg/mL.

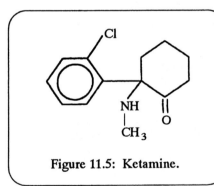

Figure 11.5: Ketamine.

Pharmacokinetics:
Ketamine may be given iv, im, po, or pr. Extensive first pass metabolism and decreased absorption necessitates the administration of higher doses when given by the oral or rectal routes. Ketamine undergoes biotransformation in the liver, yielding eight metabolites. The most significant metabolite is norketamine (also known as Metabolite I), which has 1/3 the potency of ketamine,

and subsequently undergoes hydoxylation, conjugation, and excretion in the liver.

Following administration, there is rapid absorption and distribution to the vessel rich group (see thiopental), with recovery of consciousness probably secondary to its redistribution to other tissues. Over 90% of an i.m. injection is bioavailable. Hepatic metabolism is required for elimination, with less than 5% of the administered drug recovered in the urine unchanged. There is a three phase exponential decline in ketamine levels with a T½ distribution of 24 seconds, a T½ redistribution of 4.7 minutes, and T½ elimination of 2.2 hours.

Mechanism of Action:
Three current theories about ketamines mechanism of action are:
1. N. Methyl Aspartate receptor theory. NMA receptors may represent a subgroup of the sigma (σ) opiate receptors (the PCP site), that block spinal pain reflexes.
2. Opiate receptor theory. Ketamine may have some affinity for opiate receptors but its effects cannot be reversed with naloxone.
3. Miscellaneous receptor theory. Ketamine interacts with muscarinic, cholinergic, and serotonergic receptors.

Ketamine was originally thought to cause a 'functional and electrophysiological dissociation between the thalamoneocortical and limbic systems'. Ketamine is a potent analgesic at subanaesthetic plasma concentrations. Its analgesic and anaesthetic effects may be due to different mechanisms, with the analgesic effects resulting from an interaction between ketamine and central or spinal opiate receptors.

CNS:
Ketamine anaesthesia produces a cataleptic state during which nystagmus as well as intact corneal and pupillary light reflexes may be observed. There is a generalized increase in muscle tone and purposeful movements, and vocalization may occur. Unpleasant dreams, hallucinations, or frank delirium may occur with ketamine, especially if the patient is young, female, and large doses of ketamine are given rapidly. The incidence of delirium is decreased with the concomitant administration of a benzodiazepine (eg. diazepam or midazolam), and by giving small doses slowly. The overall incidence of delirium in the 15 to 35 year old population is approximately 20%.

Intracranial pressure is not increased with ketamine provided ventilation is adequate. Intraocular pressure may or may not increase with ketamine.

RESP:
Ketamine provides general anaesthesia while preserving laryngeal and pharyngeal airway reflexes. Despite this, there are reports of pulmonary aspiration of gastric contents during ketamine anaesthesia when an artificial airway is not used. Ketamine is associated with mild respiratory depression in healthy patients following 2 mg/kg intravenously. The CO_2 response curve is shifted to the left with its slope unchanged (similar to opiates). Func-

tional residual capacity (FRC), minute ventilation (V_E), and tidal volume (V_T), are preserved as is hypoxic pulmonary vasoconstriction (HPV). In dogs, ketamine is as effective as halothane or enflurane in preventing bronchospasm. Changes in the respiratory pattern may be observed with periods of prolonged apnea, resulting in hypoxic episodes. Increased secretions occur with ketamine, and can be limited with the prior administration of an anticholinergic, such as atropine or glycopyrrolate.

CVS:
Ketamine produces both a central sympathetic stimulation and a direct negative ionotropic effect on the heart. The central sympathetic stimulation results in an increase in HR, BP, SVR, pulmonary artery pressures (PAP), coronary blood flow (CBF) and myocardial oxygen uptake (MVO2). Pulmonary vascular resistance (PVR) is unchanged if ventilation is controlled. If the normal sympathetic nervous system is blocked or exhausted, ketamine may cause direct myocardial depression.

GI:
Anorexia, nausea, and vomiting are minimal.

GU/Placenta/Fetus:
Placental transfer does occur, but neonatal depression has not been observed if the ketamine dose is limited to ≤ 1 mg/kg.

MSK:
At the neuromuscular junction, there is an increase in skeletal muscle tone, and the effects of muscle relaxants, such as succinylcholine and curare, are enhanced by ketamine.

ENDO:
Ketamine's sympathetic stimulation will result in an increase in blood glucose, plasma cortisol, and heart rate.

Dosage:
im: 5 - 10 mg/kg
iv: 1 - 2 mg/kg (To limit the risk of delirium following ketamine, it should be injected at a rate of ≤ 40 mg/minute).

Intramuscular injections in children of 9 - 13 mg/kg produce surgical anaesthesia within 3 - 4 minutes with a duration of 20 - 25 minutes. Peak plasma levels are reached approximately 15 minutes following an im injection. With iv administration a dissociated state is noted in 15 seconds, and intense analgesia, amnesia and unconsciousness occur within 45 - 60 seconds. A dose of 1 - 2 mg/kg will produce unconsciousness for 10 - 15 minutes, analgesia for 40 minutes, and amnesia for 1 - 2 hours. Subsequent iv doses of 1/3 to 1/2 the initial dose may be required.

Indications for ketamine*:
1. Sole anaesthetic for diagnostic and surgical procedures.
2. For induction of anaesthesia prior to the use of other anaesthetic agents.
3. To supplement regional anaesthetic or local anaesthetic techniques.
4. For anaesthetic induction in the severe asthmatic patient or the patient with cardiovascular collapse requiring emergency surgery.

Contraindications to ketamine:
1. Lack of knowledge of the drug.
2. Lack of resuscitative equipment.
3. Inability to maintain a patent airway.
4. Allergy or hypersensitivity to ketamine.
5. History of psychosis.
6. Cerebrovascular disease.
7. Patients for whom hypertension is hazardous.
  (eg. severe hypertension, aneurysms, heart failure, etc.)

Other side effects and toxicity:
Respiratory depression may occur and should be managed with ventilatory support. Ketamine has a wide margin of safety, and in cases of relative overdoses (up to 10 times the usual dose) there has been a protracted though complete recovery.

Other adjuvant intravenous anaesthetic agents:

Benzodiazepines: Features which result in the popularity of benzodiazepines as adjuvant intravenous anaesthetic agents include:

1. Ability to produce amnesia.
2. Minimal cardiorespiratory depressant effects.
3. Anticonvulsant activity.
4. Low incidence of tolerance and dependence.

Benzodiazepines inhibit the actions of glycine and facilitate the actions of the inhibitory neurotransmitter gamma aminobutyric acid (GABA). Benzodiazepines antianxiety and skeletal muscle relaxant effects are due to an increase in the concentration of a glycine inhibitory neurotransmitter. Facilitation of the effects of GABA results in the sedative and anticonvulsant effects of benzodiazepines. Benzodiazepines are highly lipid soluble and highly protein bound. In patients with reduced albumen levels (e.g., cirrhosis, renal insufficiency, malnutrition), the decreased plasma binding may result in an increase in free drug concentration, and an increase in drug related toxicity.

Benzodiazepines are metabolized in the liver by hepatic microsomal enzymes. The metabolites are conjugated with glucuronic acid and excreted by the kidneys. Elimination half times range from 1 - 4 hours for midazolam (Versed®), to 10 - 20 hours for lorazepam (Ativan®), and 21 - 37 hours for diazepam (Valium®).

Midazolam and diazepam are the two most commonly used benzodiazepines during operative procedures.

Midazolam (Versed®):
Midazolam's most common use intraoperatively is to provide intravenous sedation, amnesia, and to reduce anxiety. A dose of 0.5 to 3 mg intravenously (up to 0.1 mg/kg) is effective for intravenous conscious sedation. Higher doses of 0.2 - 0.4 mg/kg may be used to induce anaesthesia. Midazolam has a more rapid onset, greater amnestic effect and less postoperative sedative effects than diazepam. Pain on injection and subsequent thrombophlebitis is less likely with midazolam than with diazepam. Midazolam's duration of action is less than diazepam's, but

almost 3 times that of thiopental. It is supplied for intravenous use as a clear liquid in concentrations of 1 to 5 mg/ml.

Diazepam:
Diazepam has 1/2 to 1/3 the potency of midazolam. A dose of 1 - 10 mg is effective for intravenous conscious sedation. Higher doses of 0.15 to 1.5 mg/kg are used to induce anaesthesia. Diazepam has a high incidence of pain on intravenous injection, as well as a high incidence of subsequent phlebitis. An emulsion of diazepam (Diazemuls®) is available and has a lower incidence of venous irritation and phlebitis. Diazemuls® contains a diazepam emulsoid of soybean oil, egg lecithin, and a glycerol solution (similar to propofol), however, it is more costly than plain diazepam.

Benzodiazepine Antagonists:
Flumazenil (Anexate®) is an imidazo-benzodiazepine that specifically antagonizes benzodiazepine's central effects by competitive inhibition. The mean elimination half life of flumazenil is approximately one hour, considerably shorter than most benzodiazepines. Hence, repeat administration or infusions may be required when benzodiazepines with a longer T½ elimination are being antagonized.

Flumazenil is supplied as a colourless liquid in a concentration of 0.1 mg per mL. The usual initial dose is 0.2 mg iv over 15 seconds. If the desired level of consciousness is not obtained within 60 seconds of administration, repeated doses of 0.1 mg can be given every minute up to a maximum of 2 mg. If sedation recurs, infusions of 0.1 to 0.4 mg/hour may be used. Flumazenil is generally well tolerated. The most common side effect is nausea, and this is seen in only 4 % of patients.

Droperidol:
Butyrophenones such as droperidol and haldol are classified as major tranquilizers. Droperidol is more commonly used in the perioperative period than is haldol, because it has a shorter duration of action, and has less significant alpha adrenergic antagonist effects so marked reductions in blood pressure are unlikely. Droperidol acts at the postsynaptic receptor sites to decrease the neurotransmitter function of dopamine. It is used in the operating suite as an antiemetic and as an adjuvant to opioid analgesia (neuroleptanalgesia). Droperidol is a powerful antiemetic, inhibiting dopaminergic receptors in the chemoreceptor trigger zone of the medulla. The usual dose of droperidol as an antiemetic is 0.25 to 2.5 mg iv. Adverse side effects are dose related.

Extrapyramidal reactions are seen in approximately 1% of patients and are due to its antagonism of dopamine. For this reason, droperidol is contraindicated in patients with known Parkinson's disease. Other adverse reactions include orthostatic hypotension, and dysphoric reactions resulting in increased anxiety and an agitated state. Abnormal sleep patterns in the first 24 hours following the administration of 1.25 mg of droperidol have been reported in healthy patients undergoing minor surgical procedures. Droperidol may be administered in higher doses with an opioid such as fentanyl to produce an anaesthetic state referred to as neuroleptanalgesia. This is characterized by a trance like immobility and an appearance of tranquility. The intense analgesia produced with neuroleptanalgesia allows a variety of minor procedures to be performed (e.g., bronchoscopy, or cystoscopy). The disadvantages of this form of anaesthesia include a prolonged central nervous system depression and postoperative dysphoric reactions. For these reasons, neuroleptanalgesia is only rarely administered today.

Notes:

CHAPTER 12

Muscle Relaxants

Neuromuscular physiology*:

The neuromuscular junction consists of:

1. A motor nerve ending with mitochondria and acetylcholine vesicles (prejunctional).
2. A synaptic cleft of 20 - 30 nm in width containing extracellular fluid.
3. A highly folded skeletal muscle membrane (postjunctional).
4. Nicotinic cholinergic receptors located on both the presynaptic (nerve) and postsynaptic (muscle) membranes.

Skeletal muscle contraction involves an intricate series of events. As a nerve impulse is generated, an action potential travels down the nerve to the neuromuscular junction (NMJ) (see figure 12.1). The action potential results in the release of acetylcholine from the nerve endings into the synaptic cleft. The acetylcholine diffuses across to the muscles nicotinic cholinergic receptors causing a change in the membranes permeability to ions. The altered membrane permeability results in a sodium and potassium flux across the muscle membrane. This flux of ions decreases the muscles transmembrane electrical potential. When the resting transmembrane potential decreases from -90 mV to -45 mV, an action potential spreads over the surface of the skeletal muscle resulting in a muscular contraction. Acetylcholine's action is rapidly (< 15 milliseconds) terminated as it diffuses away from the muscles end plate, and is hydrolysed by acetylcholinesterase.

Muscle relaxants produce skeletal muscle paralysis by interfering with acetylcholine at the neuromuscular junction. Fortunately, involuntary muscles such as the heart are not affected by neuromuscular blocking drugs.

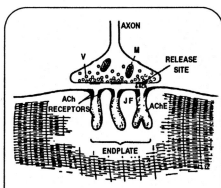

Figure 12.1: The neuromuscular junction. Ach = Acetylcholine; AChE = acetylcholinesterase; JF = junctional folds; M = mitochondria; V = Vesicle. (With permission from Drachman DB; Myasthenia gravis. N Engl J Med 298:136-142, 1978).

Classification*:

Muscle relaxants may be classified according to their duration of action (short, intermediate, or long), and on the basis of the type of neuromuscular block they produce. A non-competitive depolarizing muscle relaxant such as succinylcholine cannot be antagonized. The termination of succinylcholine's activity is dependent on hydrolysis by plasma cholinesterase. All other currently used muscle relaxants are competitive non-depolarizing agents. Their activity does not result in depolarization of the motor end-plate or muscle fibre, and their action can be reversed by the administration of an anticholinesterase agent such as neostigmine or edrophonium.

Choice of muscle relaxant:

Considerations for choosing a muscle relaxant include*:
1. Duration of action of relaxant, and duration of required muscle relaxation.
2. Route of excretion.
3. Tendency to release histamine.
4. Cardiopulmonary side effects resulting from administration. Potential adverse reactions include bradycardia, tachycardia, bronchospasm and hypotension.
5. The ability to reverse the neuromuscular block.
6. Cost.
7. Contraindications to any specific muscle relaxant.

Table 12.1 summarizes the duration of action of some commonly used muscle relaxants, and the extent to which they depend on renal excretion.

Non Depolarizing Muscle Relaxants:

Non-depolarizing neuromuscular blocking drugs compete with acetylcholine for the cholinergic nicotinic receptor. As the concentration of muscle relaxant increases at the NMJ, the intensity of muscle paralysis increases. Anticholinesterase agents inhibit the break down of acetylcholine. This results in an increase in the concentration of acetylcholine at the NMJ. Anaesthesiologists exploit this pharmacological action by administering acetylcholinesterase agents such as neostigmine and edrophonium to competitively 'reverse' the effects of a non-depolarizing neuromuscular blockade.

Mivacurium: Mivacurium is a new short-acting non-depolarizing neuromuscular blocking drug which, like succinylcholine undergoes hydrolysis by plasma cholinesterase. Patients who have deficiencies in the quality or quantity of plasma cholinesterase will have a prolonged duration of action with both mivacurium and succinylcholine (see succinylcholine, p.93). The effective dose to produce a 95% reduction in the twitch height (ED_{95}) is 0.08 mg/kg (see chapter 10: Monitoring Neuromuscular Function). Intubation with a non-depolarizing muscle relaxant is typically accomplished by the administration of 2 to 3 times the ED_{95}. Intubation with mivacurium can be performed approximately 2 - 2.5 minutes after administering twice the ED_{95}. With rapid injection of an intubating dose of mivacurium, a transient fall in blood pressure may be observed secondary to the release of histamine. Special infusion pumps are

Brand Name (Trade Name) Concentration	Block	Duration (mins.)	% dependent on renal excretion	Time to intubation (90%block) at 2 x ED$_{95}$	Intubating Dose (mg/kg)
Succinylcholine (Anectine) 20 mg/ml	Non Competitive (Depolarizing)	Short 5 - 10	0	< 60 sec	1 - 2
Mivacurium (Mivacron) 2mg/ml	Competitive Non - Depolarizing	25 - 30	0	2 - 3 min	0.16 - .30
Vecuronium (Norcuron) 10 mg/vial		Inter- mediate 45 - 60	10 - 25	2.5 - 3 min	.07 - 0.10
Rocuronium (Zemuron) 10 mg/ml		30 - 45	25	~ 80 secs	0.6
Cisatracurium (Nimbex) 10 mg/ml		20 - 60	0	3.3 min	0.1
Pancuronium (Pavulon) 1 - 2 mg/ml		Long 60 - 75	60 - 80	3 - 8 min	.06 - .10
Doxacurium (Nuromax) 1 mg/ml		50 - 130	60 - 80	3 - 10 min	0.05

Table 12.1: Properties of neuromuscular blocking agents.

frequently utilized in the operating room to deliver opioid analgesics, sedatives, or muscle relaxants. These pumps allow for both continuous infusions and bolus doses to be administered. Continuous infusions of 5 - 10 mcg/kg/min of mivacurium may be used to maintain a stable neuromuscular blockade during the procedure.

Cisatracurium: Cisatracurium is classified as an intermediate-acting neuromuscular blocking drug, and is one of 10 isolated isomer of it's predescesor atracurium. It undergoes hydrolysis in the plasma by a non-enzymatic process referred to as Hoffman elimination, and by an ester hydrolysis reaction. Significant histamine release resulting in hypotension, tachycardia, and bronchospasm, that may occur after rapid administration of atracurium is not seen with cisatracurium. This lack of histamine release is the main advantage of cisatracurium over it's parent compound atracurium. The ED_{95} of cisatracurium is 0.05 mg/kg. A stable neuromuscular block can be achieved using an infusion of cisatracurium at a rate of 1 - 5 mcg/kg/min. Cisatracurium is an ideal agent for patients with renal or hepatic insufficiency requiring muscle relaxation.

Vecuronium: Vecuronium is an intermediate-acting neuromuscular blocking agent. It is a popular agent because it does not produce any undesirable cardiovascular side effects even when administered rapidly in large doses. Its ED_{95} is 0.05 mg/kg. The onset time for neuromuscular relaxation following 2 x the ED_{95} is 150 - 200 seconds. This can be shortened by the administration of a small 'priming' dose (0.01 mg/kg) of vecuronium, followed by 2 - 4 times the ED_{95}. This can achieve conditions suitable for intubation in approximately 90 seconds from the time of administration. The duration of neuromuscular block will be increased to more than 1 hour if a larger dose is used for intubation. Continuous infusions of 0.5 - 1.5 mcg/kg/min have been used to maintain a stable neuromuscular block during the procedure.

Rocuronium: This new intermediate acting non-depolarizing neuromuscular relaxant may replace atracurium, vecuronium, and mivacurium as the relaxant of choice for short and intermediate procedures. It has just recently been released, and has a duration of action, route of metabolism, and lack of hemodynamic side-effects similar to that of vecuronium. Rocuronium's major ad-vantage is it's ability to quickly induce a neuromuscular block, making it suitable for a rapid induction and intubation sequence. It has an ED_{95} of approximately 0.3 mg/kg. The onset time (i.e. time to 90% depression of T1 twitch height) for an intubating dose of rocuronium (i.e. 2 x ED_{95}) is 60 - 80 seconds. By contrast, vecuronium has a much slower onset time of 150 - 200 seconds. Rocuronium's onset time is comparable to the onset time following 1.5 mg/kg of succinylcholine (50 - 70 seconds). Hence, rocuronium matches succinylcholine's onset time, and avoids its potential side effects. Nevertheless, it must be remembered that the duration of action of this dose of succinylcholine is only 8 - 12 minutes, compared to 35 - 45 minutes for rocuronium. Continuous infusions in the range of 4 - 16 mcg/kg/min. can be used to maintain a stable neuromuscular block. This should be reduced by 30 - 50% when administered in the presence of 1% isoflurane (similar to all other neuromuscular relaxants).

Pancuronium: Pancuronium is a long-acting neuromuscular blocking drug. Administration of pancuronium is frequently associated with a modest (< 15%) increase in heart rate, blood pressure, and cardiac output. The increase in heart rate is due to its blockade of the cardiac muscarinic receptors, as well as an inhibition of catecholamine reuptake by sympathetic nerves. Pancuronium administration does not result in histamine release. The ED_{95} of pancuronium is 0.06 mg/kg. Pancuronium is much more dependent on renal excretion than the other clinically used muscle relaxants. A prolonged neuromuscular block will result when pancuronium is administered to patients with renal failure or insufficiency.

d - Tubocurare: The muscle paralyzing properties of curare were well know to South American natives who used this drug to immobilize and kill animals with blowgun darts. In 1942 Griffith and Johnson in Montreal introduced the medical world to the paralyzing properties of curare. Since the early 1990's curare has been unavailable in Canada, and is now only of historical interest. In the 1980's curare was most frequently used to attenuate the muscle fasciculations and postoperative myalgias associated with the administration of succinylcholine. A small 'pretreatment' dose of curare (3 mg per 70kg) was administered approximately 3 minutes prior to the administration of succinylcholine, and was appreciated for it's excellent 'defasciculating' properties. Today, anesthesiologists who wish to attenuate the muscle fasculations and postop myalgia's seen with succinylcholine administer a small (~ 1/10 intubating dose) of a non-depolarizing muscle relaxant 3 minutes prior to succinylchole (eg., rocuronium 5 mg per 70 kg).

Depolarizing Muscle Relaxants:
Succinylcholine is the most frequently used muscle relaxant that is administered outside the operating room by a non-anaesthetist physician. Hence a detailed discussion of its properties is included in this chapter. Succinylcholine is the only depolarizing neuromuscular blocking agent that is clinically used. Depolarizing muscle relaxants *bind and depolarize* the endplate cholinergic receptors. By contrast, non-depolarizing muscle relaxants competitively block the action of acetylcholine. The initial depolarization can be observed as irregular, generalized fasciculations occurring in the skeletal muscles.

Succinylcholine (Anectine®)
Classification:
Non-competitive depolarizing neuromuscular blocking agent.

Physical-Chemical Properties:
Succinylcholine physically resembles two acetylcholine molecules linked end to end. It has two quaternary ammonium cations which interact with the anionic sites on the muscle end plate receptors.

Ninety percent of succinylcholine undergoes hydrolysis by plasma cholinesterase (psuedocholinesterase) before it reaches the neuromuscular junction. After binding to the end plate muscle receptors and causing skeletal muscle relaxation, it diffuses out of the NMJ. Outside the NMJ, succinylcholine is again exposed to plasma cholinesterase and the remaining 10% is hydrolysed. The metabolites of succinylcholine are excreted in the urine. Peak effect is reached within 60 seconds of administration, and the neuro-muscular blocking effects of succinyl-choline typically dissipate over the next 5 to 10 minutes.

Phase I and Phase II Blocks:

Succinylcholine produces a 'prolonged acetylcholine (Ach) effect'. It combines with the Ach receptor to depolarize the end plate, resulting in a generalized depolarization (seen as succinylcholine induced fasciculations). The membrane remains depolarized and unresponsive until succinylcholine diffuses away from the endplate (due to a concentration gradient). This initial neuromuscular block is referred to as a phase I block. If large amounts of succinylcholine are given (eg. 4 - 6 mg/kg), a different neuro-muscular block may occur. This block is referred to as a phase II block. Clinically this may occur when repeated doses of succinylcholine are given, or when succinylcholine infusions are used. A phase II block has features which resemble a neuromuscular block that is produced by non-depolarizing muscle relaxants. The actual mechanism of a phase II block is unknown.

Characteristics of Phase I Blocks:

1. Similar response to a single twitch
2. No post-tetanic facilitation
3. Train of four (TOF) ratio > 0.7
4. Muscle fasciculations prior to paralysis
5. Decreased amplitude, but sustained response to tetanic stimulus
6. The neuromuscular block is increased when cholinesterase inhibitors are administered

Characteristics of Phase II Blocks:

1. Decreased response to a single twitch
2. Post-tetanic facilitation present
3. Train of four (TOF) ratio < 0.7
4. No fasciculations with onset of paralysis

5. Response to a tetanus stimulus fades during the stimulus
6. The neuromuscular block can be reversed with anticholinesterase agents

The presence of a normal amount of active plasma cholinesterase is essential to terminate the effects of succinylcholine. In certain conditions, the levels of plasma cholinesterase may be low, and this is referred to as a quantitative decrease in cholinesterase levels. The consequences of a low plasma cholinesterase level are generally of little significance. In patients with severe liver disease with plasma cholinesterase levels as low as 20% of normal, the duration of a neuromuscular block resulting from the administration of succinylcholine increases threefold (eg. 5 to 15 minutes). Liver disease, cancer, pregnancy, and certain drugs such as cyclophosphamide, phenylzine, and monoamine oxidase inhibitors have all been associated with low cholinesterase levels.

Abnormalities in plasma cholinesterase activity are inherited. Patients may have normal plasma levels of cholinesterase, with a severely impaired enzyme activity. This is referred to as a qualitative decrease in plasma cholinesterase. Plasma cholinesterase enzyme activity is genetically determined by four alleles identified as the silent or absent allele (s), the usual allele (u), the dibucaine allele (d), and the fluoride allele (f). The normal plasma cholinesterase genotype is EuEu. Patients with abnormal cholinesterase activity are otherwise healthy and can be identified only by a specific blood test that identifies the genotype and enzyme activity. The sixteen possible genotypes are expressed as ten possible phenotypes. Six of these ten phenotypes are associated with a marked reduction in the hydrolysis of succinylcholine. Patients with the genotype EaEa have a marked reduction in the hydrolysis of succinylcholine. These patients will have a prolonged neuromuscular block that can be increased from ten minutes to several hours following a normal intubating dose of 1 - 2 mg/kg of succinylcholine. The EaEa genotype has a frequency of approximately 1:3200.

The treatment of postoperative paralysis secondary to deficiencies in plasma cholinesterase activity includes controlled ventilation, reassurance, and sedation. Blood samples should be taken to confirm the diagnosis and identify the enzyme genotype. Immediate family members should be tested to determine their genotypes and susceptibility. Medical alert bracelets should be worn by any patient with a significant reduction in their plasma cholinesterase activity.

Pharmacodynamics:
CNS:
Succinylcholine has no known effect on consciousness, pain threshold or cerebral function. An increase in intraocular pressure (IOP) begins within 1 min of administration of succinylcholine. A peak rise in IOP of 6-10 mmHg occurs at 2-4 minutes, and subsides by 6 minutes. Factors that may increase IOP include: an increase in central venous pressure, changes in pH, $PaCO_2$, mean arterial pressure, and a direct effect from the extraocular muscles. A normal IOP is 10 - 20 mmHg. An increase in IOP under anaesthesia is undesirable in patients with an injury that disrupts the globe's integrity. These patients are at risk of vitreous extrusion and damage to the eye if the IOP increases. While succinylcholine increases IOP, crying, straining, or coughing can result in much greater increases of up to 50 mmHg. Increases in intracranial pressure (ICP) of up to 10 mmHg may occur following succinylcholine administration. The mechanism of the increase in ICP is thought to be due to the central mobilization of blood that results from succinylcholine's generalized muscle contractions.

RESP:
A progressive paralysis from eyelids to the jaw, limbs, abdominal, intercostal and diaphragmatic muscles follows the administration of succinylcholine.

CVS:
Succinylcholine stimulates both the nicotinic and muscarinic cholinergic autonomic receptors. As a consequence of muscarinic cholinergic stimulation, bradycardia, dysrhythmias, and sinus arrest may be observed. This vagal response is prominent among children and, after repeated doses, in adults. It may be inhibited with anticholinergics such as atropine.

GI:
Succinylcholine iincreases the intragastric in proportion to the intensity of the muscle fasciculations in the abdo-

men. It can be limited with prior use of non-depolarizing muscle relaxant.

GU:
Succinylcholine does not rely on renal excretion. It's metabolites, succinic acid and choline, however, are excreted by the kidney. Patients with renal failure may have pre-existing hyperkalemia, and may be susceptible to succinylcholine-induced hyperkalemia.

The usual serum potassium response following succinylcholine is a transient and brief increase in the extracellular K+ concentration of ~ 0.5 meq/L. Generally patients with K+ concentrations of ≥ 5.5 meq/L should not receive succinylcholine, and all but emergency procedures should be delayed. Succinylcholine does not cross the placenta because of its low fat solubility and its ionized state.

MSK:
Succinylcholine has no direct effect on the uterus or other smooth muscles. Myalgias following the administration of succinylcholine are infrequent in children, the geriatric population, and pregnant patients. The incidence of succinylcholine myalgias can be decreased with prior administration of a non-depolarizing muscle relaxant such as curare (3 mg/70kg). Fasciculations result in the release of myoglobin into the serum (myoglobinemia). The excretion of myoglobin into the urine (myoglobinuria) is more common in children, and can be decreased with prior treatment with non-depolarizing muscle relaxants. Succinylcholine increases the masseter muscle tone in the jaw. Some patients may respond with an abnormally high tone in masseter muscle following succinylcholine. These patients are said to have developed a masseter muscle spasm, and may represent a subgroup of patients susceptible to malignant hyperthermia.

Hyperkalemia following succinylcholine**:
A few cholinergic receptors are located along skeletal muscle membranes outside of the NMJ. The receptors are called extrajunctional cholinergic receptors. The numbers of these receptors increase dramatically over a period of 24 hours whenever nerve impulse activity to the muscle is interrupted. Acute disruption of nerve activity to skeletal muscle occurs in patients who have sustained third degree burns or traumatic paralysis (paraplegia, quadriplegia). Administration of succinylcholine to these patients will result in an abnormally high flux of potassium out of the muscle cells because of the increased number of receptors. An acute rise in the serum potassium to levels as high as 13 meq/L following succinylcholine may result in sudden cardiac arrest. Succinylcholine is absolutely contraindicated in these patients. The administration of a non-depolarizing muscle relaxant in these patients does not result in a hyperkalemic response because the receptors are simply blocked and not depolarized.

Patients who are at risk of a hyper-kalemic response following the administration of succinylcholine include:

1. Patients with extensive *third degree burns.* Succinylcholine should be avoided if the injury is more than 24 hours old, and for 6 months following the healing of the burn injury.
2. Patients with *nerve damage or neuromuscular diseases* such as muscular dystrophy are susceptible to hyperkalemia and cardiac standstill with succinylcholine. The degree of hyperkalemia appears to be related to the degree and extent of muscle affected.
3. Severe intra-abdominal *infections.*
4. Severe *closed head injury.*
5. *Upper motor neuron lesions.*

Specific Diseases:

1. *Myasthenia Gravis* - All muscle relaxants are best avoided, if possible, in patients with myasthenia gravis. These patients behave as if partially curarized. They are very sensitive to non-depolarizing muscle relaxants, and may be sensitive or resistant to depolarizing muscle relaxants.

2. *Myasthenic Syndrome:* The Eaton-Lambert Syndrome is a proximal muscle myopathy associated with a carcinoma of the bronchus. Unlike myasthenia gravis, muscle fatigue decreases with exercise, and the eyelids are less affected. These patients are unusually sensitive to both depolarizing and non-depolarizing muscle relaxants.

3. *Myotonia:* Patients with myotonia congenita, myotonia dystrophica, and paramyotonia congenita may all develop a severe, generalized contracture if given succinylcholine. The use of a depolarizing muscle relaxant such as succinylcholine in these patients may result in a secondary generalized contracture of the skeletal muscles, and prevent airway maintenance and ventilation.

4. *Familial Periodic Paralysis:* Succinylcholine can precipitate a generalized contracture and should be avoided in these patients.

Dosage & Administration:
Intubating dose:
With curare pretreatment:
1.5 - 2 mg/kg intravenously:

Without curare pretreatment:
1 - 1.5 mg/kg iv.

Infusion:
An infusion may be used for short procedures to maintain a stable neuromuscular block. Recommended rates for infusion are 50 - 150 mcg/kg/min.

Indications:
1. Skeletal muscle relaxation during endotracheal intubation
2. Abdominal operations of short duration
3. Prior to electroconvulsive therapy (ECT), to prevent the possibility of seizure induced injury (e.g., vertebral fracture)
4. Emergency treatment for laryngospasm

Contraindications** :

Absolute
1. Inability to maintain an airway
2. Lack of resuscitative equipment
3. Known hypersensitivity or allergy
4. Positive history of Malignant Hyperthermia
5. Myotonia (M.Congenita, M. Dystrophica or Paramyotonia congenita)
6. Patients identified as being at risk of a hyperkalemic response to succinylcholine (see above).

Relative:
1. Known history of plasma cholinesterase deficiency
2. Myasthenia Gravis
3. Myasthenic Syndrome
4. Familial Periodic Paralysis
5. Open eye injury

Reversal of neuromuscular blockade:
Muscle relaxation produced by non-depolarizing neuromuscular agents may be "reversed" by anticholinesterase agents such as edrophonium and neostigmine. These agents prevent the breakdown of acetylcholine in the NMJ. The increased concentration of acetylcholine at the NMJ competes with the muscle relaxant allowing the receptor once again to become responsive to the release of acetylcholine from the nerves.

The increased concentrations of acetylcholine also stimulate the muscarinic cholinergic receptors, resulting in bradycardia, salivation, and increased bowel peristalsis. Anticholinergic agents such as atropine and glycopyrrolate are administered prior to reversal, to block these unwanted muscarinic effects. Common combinations of anticholinergic and anticholinesterase agents used to reverse a neuromuscular block are atropine 0.01 mg/kg with edrophonium (Tensilon®) 0.5 - 1.0 mg/kg, or glycopyrrolate 0.01 mg/kg with neostigmine (Prostigmin®) 0.05 - 0.07 mg/kg intravenously.

Timing of reversal:
There are numerous methods of assessing the depth of neuromuscular blockade. The most common of these include the train of four (TOF) stimulus, tetanus stimulus, and the train of four (TOF) ratio. The train of four stimulus (TOF) applies four brief electrical stimuli of 2 Hz each over a period of 2 seconds. The train of four ratio, (T4/T1), is the ratio of the twitch response of the fourth stimulus (T4) to the first stimulus (T1). In most circumstances, adequate muscle relaxation for surgery occurs when only one of the four twitches is observed. This corresponds to a ≥ 90% blockade of the NMJ receptors. One must consider the intensity and anticipated duration of neuromuscular block before attempting to antagonize it. Reversal may be unsuccessful if only one of the four twitches is present. With inadequate reversal of muscle relaxation, the patient will have a weak hand grip, be unable to cough effectively, and unable to sustain lifting their head from their pillow for 5 seconds. Treatment of inadequate reversal includes supportive ventilation, sedation, analgesia, and adequate time for the neuromuscular block to dissipate.

CHAPTER 13

Inhalational Anaesthetic Agents

The intravenous anaesthetic agents introduced in chapter 11 (propofol, ketamine, and thiopentothal) are frequently used to induce the anaesthetic state. To maintain the anaesthetic state, volatile anaesthetic agents are commonly vaporized and delivered to the patient through the anaesthetic machine and anaesthetic circuit. This volatile vapour is then delivered to the lungs where it diffuses across the alveolar capillary membrane and is dissolved in the blood. The blood then carries it to the brain and other organs in the body.

Intravenous drugs are typically delivered according to a specific number of milligrams or micrograms per kilogram of body tissue. Inhalational agents on the other hand are administered according to a specific concentration. The concentration of a gas is expressed as a percentage of the volume of anaesthetic gas to the total volume of the gas mixture. For example if we deliver 2 liters/min. of oxygen and 4 liters/min. of nitrous oxide (N_2O) to a patient, the concentration of N_2O is $4/(2 + 4) = 66\%$. If we want to add a 1% concentration of isoflurane to this mixture we would have to add approximately 60 ml of a saturated isoflurane vapour to the 6 liters of fresh gas flow (0.01×6000 ml $= 60$ ml). Modern anaesthetic vaporizers are able to vaporize liquid inhalational anaesthetic agents such that very accurate concentrations can be delivered to the patient by simply setting the vaporizer dial at the desired concentration.

The role of inhalational anaesthetic drugs in current anaesthetic practice is changing. The introduction of potent intravenous agents, including muscle relaxants, opioids, benzodiazepines, propofol, and intravenous infusion techniques have decreased the need for high doses of inhalational agents. In anaesthesia, a number of different agents representing different classes of drugs are chosen to minimize the side effects of any one agent and capitalize on each agent's benefits.

Inhalational agents are compared to one another according to their minimal alveolar concentration** or "MAC" values. The MAC value of an inhalational agent is the alveolar concentration in oxygen at one atmosphere of pressure that will prevent 50% of the subjects from making a purposeful movement in response to a painful stimulus such as a surgical incision. The MAC value can be considered the effective dose in 50% of the subjects or the ED_{50}. Knowledge of the MAC value allows one to compare the potencies of different inhalational agents. The MAC values of dif-

Table 13.1: Factors which alter anaesthetic requirements (MAC).

Increased MAC	No change in MAC	Decreased MAC

Hyperthermia
Chronic drug
  abuse: Ethanol
Acute use of
  amphetamines
Hyperthyroidism
	Gender
	Duration of anaesthesia
	Carbon dioxide tensions:
	  $PaCO_2$ 21 - 95 mmHg
	Metabolic acid-base status
	Hypertension
		Increasing age
		Hypothermia
		Severe hypotension
		Other anaesthetic agents:
		  opioids, benzodiazepines
		Acute drug intoxication:
		  Ethanol
		Pregnancy
		Hypothyroidism
		Other drugs:
		  clonidine, reserpine

ferent anaesthetic agents are additive. Nitrous oxide is the only inhalational agent that is routinely combined with another inhalational agent such as iso-flurane, enflurane, or halothane. It is necessary to establish an anaesthetic depth equivalent to 1.2 to 1.3 of the MAC value. The added 20 - 30% MAC depth of anaesthesia will prevent movement in 95% of patients. The MAC value of N_2O is 105%, which is approximately one-hundred-fold greater than the other inhalational agents. Because the recommended minimum concentration of oxygen delivered during general anaesthesia is 30%, the maximum concentration on N_2O is 70% (approximately 0.7 MAC). Hence, nitrous oxide alone is unable to provide adequate anaesthesia. Opioid analgesics, benzodiazepines, or other inhalational agents may be added to supplement the nitrous oxide. Table 13.1 lists factors that increase or decrease the MAC values. Table 13.2 lists differences in inhalational agents as well as their MAC values, with and without nitrous oxide.

The rapidity with which the anaesthetic state is reached depends on how quickly the anaesthetic inhalational agent reaches the brain to exert its partial pressure effects.

Factors determining how quickly the inhalational agent reaches the alveoli include:
1. The inspired concentration of anaesthetic gas being delivered by the anaesthetic machine (concentration effect).
2. The gas flow rate through the anaesthetic machine.
3. The amount of alveolar ventilation (V_A = Respiratory Rate x Tidal Volume).

Increasing any of these factors will result in a faster rise in the alveolar concentration of the inhalational agent.

Factors determining how quickly the inhalational agent reaches the brain from the alveoli in order to establish anaesthesia include:
1. The rate of blood flow to the brain.
2. The solubility of the inhalational agent in the brain.

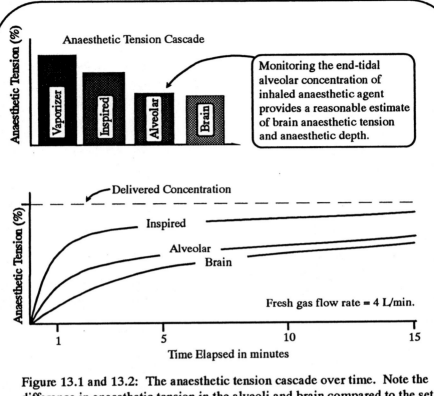

Figure 13.1 and 13.2: The anaesthetic tension cascade over time. Note the difference in anaesthetic tension in the alveoli and brain compared to the set vaporizer concentration being delivered. Increasing either the fresh gas flow rate or anaesthetic concentration will result in a faster delivery of the inhaled anaesthetic agent to the brain.

3. The difference in the arterial and venous concentrations of the inhalational agent.

Increasing any of these factors will hasten the onset of anaesthesia.

Patients with low cardiac output states (eg. shock states) may have a rapid rise in the alveolar partial pressure of an inhalational anaesthetic agent. This will result in a more rapid onset in anaesthesia, with possible exaggerated cardiorespiratory depressant effects.

The cascade of anaesthetic partial pressures starts at the vaporizer. The gas from the vaporizer is diluted by exhaled gas to form the inspired gas. With a circle system, a fresh gas flow of 4 - 5 liters per minute will raise the inspired anaesthetic tension close to the vaporizer's delivered concentration. As the body continues to take up the inhaled anaesthetic gas, the alveolar anaesthetic tension will remain below the inspired anaesthetic tension for many hours. The brain can be considered the final step in the anaesthetic cascade. The brain tension will approach the alveolar tension within 8 to 10 minutes of any change. Monitoring the alveolar end-tidal concentration of the inhaled anaesthetic agent provides a reasonable estimate of the brain anaesthetic tension (see figure 13.1 and 13.2).

Nitrous Oxide:

Nitrous oxide is an inert, inorganic, colourless, tasteless, and odourless gas. It has a rapid onset and a quick recovery of 3 to 10 minutes due to its low solubility in blood. Its low potency (MAC = 105%) limits the amount that can be administered, and its usefulness when high concentrations of oxygen are required. Myocardial depression is usually minimal in healthy patients, however significant cardiovascular depression may occur in patients with coexisting myocardial dysfunction or in patients in a shock state.

Nitrous oxide is 34 times more soluble than nitrogen. This property results in three special anaesthetic phenomena. At the beginning of anaesthesia, N2O leaves the alveoli much faster than nitrogen can leave the body tissues to fill the space left by N2O. The result is an increase in the concentration of other gases in the alveoli (oxygen, and other inhalational agents). This increase in concentration speeds the onset in inhalational anaesthetic effect, and is referred to as the **second gas effect**.

Diffusion hypoxia may result at the end of the anaesthetic. As nitrous oxide is discontinued, the body stores of nitrous oxide are released and flood the alveoli, diluting the oxygen present in the alveoli. When only room air is administered at the end of the anaesthetic, the dilution of oxygen may be sufficient to create a hypoxic mixture, and result in hypoxemia. Other factors contributing to hypoxemia at the end of anaesthesia include respiratory depression due to anaesthetic agents, residual neuromuscular blockade, and pain with splinted respirations. The administration of 100% oxygen at the end of an anaesthetic may avoid hypoxemia resulting from any of these causes.

Finally, closed air spaces will expand in the presence of nitrous oxide due to the differences in solubility of nitrogen and nitrous oxide. With the administration of 66% N2O, a closed air space will expand 2 times in volume over a period of approximately 15 minutes. For this reason N2O is contraindicated in patients with a pneumothorax, closed loop bowel obstruction, air embolism, or any other closed air space in the body.

Nitrous oxide undergoes very little metabolism and is excreted unchanged by the lungs.

The most commonly used inhalational agents today are nitrous oxide, isoflurane, enflurane, and halothane. The latter three are synthetic, colourless liquids that are non flammable and administered as a vapour from a vaporizer on the anaesthesia machine. A dose-related depression of cardiorespiratory function is common to each of these inhalational agents. All three produce smooth muscle relaxation, and this property has been exploited to produce bronchodilation in patients with status asthmaticus, and uterine relaxation in patients with a retained placenta. Halothane, enflurane, and isoflurane are all contraindicated in patients with malignant hyperthermia.

Isoflurane:

Isoflurane is the most common inhalational agent used for adult anaesthesia in North America. It has a MAC value of 1.16%, and has the fastest uptake and washout times of these three inhalational agents. It is not as well tolerated as halothane for an inhalational anaesthetic induction because of its pungent odour and tendency to irritate the airways. These irritating effects may result in coughing and breath-holding if isoflurane is administered too quickly. Isoflurane is the preferred agent for neurosurgical procedures as it causes the least increase in cerebral blood flow and intracranial pressure. Isoflurane has the least depressant effect on the myocardium. The reduction in blood pressure is accompanied by a similar reduction in vascular resistance such that there is little change in cardiac output. In certain patients (especially young healthy patients), isoflurane may produce a significant sinus tachycardia. In a small percentage of patients with coronary artery disease, isoflurane may cause vasodilation of the distal endocardial vessels, and result in a 'coronary steal'. A coronary steal is produced when blood is diverted away from the collateral dependent ischemic regions of the heart to the areas of vasodilation. The significance of this observation is still debated.

Halothane:

Halothane is the agent of choice for an inhalational anaesthetic induction, and is the most common inhalational agent used in paediatric anaesthesia. Halothane decreases myocardial contractility, slows the heart rate, and decreases cardiac conduction. The myocardium is sensitized to catecholamines in the presence of halothane, resulting in severe ventricular dysrhythmias if the body releases catecholamines (stress), or if exogenous catecholamines such as epinephrine are administered. Cerebral blood flow increases secondary to cerebral vasodilation and may result in an undesired increase in intracranial pressure.

Halothane's popularity in adult anaesthesia has declined because of its implication in causing postoperative hepatitis. "Halothane hepatitis" is believed to occur in approximately 1 in 10,000 halothane anaesthetics and presents as postoperative fever, jaundice, eosinophilia, and occasionally extensive hepatic necrosis and death. Hepatitis following isoflurane and enflurane exposure is very rare, as is hepatitis in the paediatric population following any inhalational agent (including halothane). There is a ten fold difference in metabolism of these three inhalational agents. The main route of excretion is through the lungs, but approximately 20% of halothane is metabolized by the liver. By contrast 2% of enflurane and only 0.2% of isoflurane undergoe metabolism by the P_{450} enzyme system. Both allergic and metabolic mechanisms may be active in producing hepatitis following

Table 13.2: Comparison of three common inhalational anaesthetic agents.

	Isoflurane	Halothane	Enflurane
MAC in Oxygen*	1.16%	0.75%	1.68%
MAC in 70% N2O	0.50%	0.29%	0.57%
CNS	Causes the lowest increase in ICP of the 3 agents when ventilation is controlled	Increases ICP and CBF.	Increases ICP. Potential to cause CNS excitation and seizures at high concentrations.
Resp.	Irritating to the airways, and more difficult to use for inhalational induction. Decreases tidal volume and minute ventilation, accompanied by an increase in the respiratory rate.	Good for inhalational inductions, and is less irritating to the airways. Decreases tidal volume, and minute ventilation, accompanied by an increase in the respiratory rate.	Depresses respiration more than halothane or isoflurane.
CVS	Increases heart rate. Decreases BP and CO. Potential to create a 'coronary steal'.	Depresses BP, HR, CO and conduction. Sensitizes the myocardium to adrenaline induced dysrhythmias.	Depresses cardiac function more than halothane or isoflurane.
Neuromuscular	Potentiates muscle relaxants	Potentiates muscle relaxants less than Isoflurane or Enflurane.	Potentiates muscle relaxants.
Metabolism	0.17%	15 - 20%	2.4%
Other	Most common agent used in adult anaesthesia.	Halothane Hepatitis association in adults. Cheapest agent of the three.	Second choice agent in adult anaesthesia in North America.

exposure to halothane. Repeated exposures to halothane over a short period of time have also been thought to contribute to halothane hepatitis in patients.

Enflurane:
Enflurane has a MAC of 1.68%, more than twice that of halothane's MAC value of 0.75%. Enflurane is a potent cardiorespiratory depressant, decreasing both respiratory drive and cardiac func-

tion to a greater extent than halothane. Unlike halothane or isoflurane, enflurane produces abnormal electroencephalographic (EEG) patterns resembling seizure activity. This is only observed in some patients during deep enflurane anaesthesia with lowered PaCO2 levels secondary to mechanical hyperventilation. Occasionally tonic clonic movements under enflurane anaesthesia have been observed. Despite the lack of documented adverse postoperative sequelae in these patients, enflurane is best avoided in patients with a history of a seizure disorder.

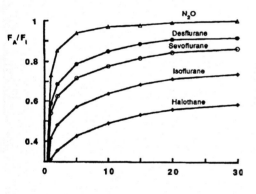

Minutes of Administration

Figure 13.3. For potent anaesthetics, solubility determines the increase in the alveolar (F_A) anaesthetic concentration toward the concentration inspired (F_I): the least soluble anaesthetic (desflurane) shows the most rapid increase; the most soluble anaesthetic (halothane) shows the least rapid increase. Reproduced with permission. Eger II, Edmond I. New Inhaled Anesthetics. Anesthesiology 80:906-922, 1994

Desflurane and Sevoflurane:
Desflurane and sevoflurane are two volatile anaesthetics which have been recently introduced in Canada. Both have low solubilities in blood, approaching that of nitrous oxide, so induction and emergence from anaesthesia is rapid. Cardiovascular, respiratory, neurological and neuromuscular effects of both agents are similar to those of isoflurane.

Desflurane is unique in that it boils at room temperature (22.8°C). Because of this physical property, desflurane requires a special heated and electronically controlled vaporizer to administer it safely. Desflurane has a MAC value in oxygen of 6% compared to sevoflurane which has a MAC value of 2% in oxygen. Desflurane has a pungent odour, and like isoflurane can cause coughing and breath holding if administered too rapidly. Sevoflurane is more pleasant smelling and is well suited for inhalational induction of anesthesia.

Sevoflurane, like enflurane, is metabolized in the liver yielding inorganic fluoride. Approximately 3% of sevoflurane is broken down in this fashion. Is is degraded by the chemicals used to absorb the patients' CO2 in their patient's breathing circuit. Production of a renal toxin called "compound A" at low fresh gas flows has lead to the recommendation that sevoflurane be administered with a minimum of two liters of fresh gas flow. In contrast, desflurane is the least metabolized of the volatile anesthetics (0.02%), and is ideally suited for use in low flow anaesthetic techniques.

Sevoflurane and Desflurane have had a major impact on our anesthetic practice. While structurally similar to their parents Halothane and Isoflurane, the substitution of a couple of key chlorine atoms with fluorine atoms results in their lower observed solubilities. This translates clinically into a more rapid induction and recovery from anesthesia.

Sevoflurane, unlike isoflurane, does not have an unpleasant smell, and is well tolerated in adults for inhalational induction of anesthesia. Using high concentrations of Sevoflurane at induction (5 - 8%, with or without nitrous oxide), the patient can be taken from an awake state to an anesthetized state with as little as one vital capacity breath. Anesthesia sufficient for laryngeal mask placement and intubation can be achieved after three to five minutes of breathing a high concentration of Sevoflurane.

Desflurane is not suitable for inhalational induction due to it's irritating and pungent properties. When given rapidly in high concentrations (6% or more) it may result in coughing, breath-holding, laryngospasm, tachycardia, and hypertension. Unlike Sevoflurane, Desflurane is essentially inert with only 0.02% undergoing metabolism. Very low fresh gas flow anesthesia can be safely practiced with Desflurane, limiting the increased cost of Desflurane when compared to Halothane and Isoflurane.

Clinical Note:
How do we know if the patient is receiving enough anaesthetic?

Our general anesthetic goals are to administer enough anaesthetic that the patient's awareness and their pain response to surgery is suppressed. Our goal is to provide adequate anaesthesia (inhibit awareness) yet at the same time avoid a relative anesthetic overdose.

We can use the knowledge that the MAC values of the individual inhalational agents are additive.

Let's assume our patient is under general anaesthesia and is receiving end-tidal concentrations of 63% nitrous oxide with 0.4% isoflurane. We can calculate the relative contributions of these inhalational agents to the patients anaesthetic.

63 % Nitrous oxide (MAC = 105 %)
$$\therefore 63/105 = \underline{0.60 \text{ MAC}}$$

0.4 % Isoflurane (MAC = 1.16 %)
$$\therefore 0.4 / 1.16 = \underline{0.35 \text{ MAC}}$$
$$\underline{0.95 \text{ MAC}}$$

As stated earlier we generally provide 1.2 - 1.3 times the MAC value to achieve adequate anaesthesia in 95% of patients. In addition to the inhalational agents this patient is receiving, he/she probably has also received a preoperative sedative, and intraoperative intravenous agents such as an opioid, benzodiazepine, and general anaesthetic induction agent (e.g., propofol). These will also contribute to the depth of anaesthesia for this patient. Repeated assessments for inadequate anaesthesia or excessive depth of anaesthesia are made during the surgery, and corresponding corrective adjustments in the anaesthetic depth are made. These are based on the patients vital signs, tearing, or obvious movement (see chapter 10; monitoring in anaesthesia).

References:

1. Miller R.D. editor. Anesthesia third edition. Churchill Livingstone Inc. 1990.
2. Barash PG, Cullen BF, Stoelting RK., editors. Clinical Anesthesia second edition. J.B. Lippincott Co., Philadelphia 1993.
3. Elliot RD. What can gas monitoring tell us? Winterlude symposium on monitoring and equipment. University of Ottawa 1994.

Notes:

CHAPTER 14

Narcotic Agonists and Antagonists

Opium is derived from the dried juice of the poppy plant, which contains over twenty plant alkaloids, including morphine, and codeine. An opiate refers to any preparation from, or derivative of, opium. A narcotic refers to any substance that produces both analgesia and stupor, and includes both opium alkaloid derivatives and synthetic analgesic compounds.

In this chapter, we shall present 5 commonly used intraoperative anaesthetic narcotics: morphine, meperidine, fentanyl, sufentanil, and alfentanil. Chapter 16 reviews other narcotic and non narcotic analgesic agents useful in managing acute postoperative pain. The properties of naloxone, a pure narcotic antagonist are presented at the end of this chapter.

Site of Action:
Opioid receptors are predominately located in the brain stem, spinal cord, and gastrointestinal tract. Narcotics exert their analgesic action by interacting with opioid receptors in the brainstem (amygdala, corpus striatum, periaqueductal gray matter, and medulla), and in the substantia gelatinosa in the spinal cord. Three classes of opioid receptors are primarily involved with

mediation of the analgesic and anaes-

μ (Mu) receptor
Analgesia, respiratory depression, euphoria, physical dependence
κ (Kappa) receptor
Analgesia, sedation, respiratory depression, miosis
σ (Sigma) receptor
Dysphoria, hallucinations, tachypnea, tachycardia

thetic properties of narcotics. The effects of stimulation of mu (μ), kappa (κ), and sigma (σ) receptors are summarized in the table below.

Features common to all narcotics include a dose related depression of respiration, sensorium, and pain perception. They are rapidly distributed through the body following intravenous injection. Hepatic metabolism is the primary route of elimination and the majority of inactive metabolites are excreted unchanged in the urine. A systems review of the other pharmacodynamic properties of narcotics is presented below.

CNS:

Opioids produce both sedation and interfere with the sensory perception of painful stimuli. Although large doses of opioids produce unconsciousness, they are generally incapable of providing complete anaesthesia, and cannot guarantee total amnesia. Dysphoric reactions rather than euphoria may occur when opioids are administered to patients who are not experiencing pain. Stimulation of the chemoreceptor trigger zone by narcotics may result in nausea and emesis.

RESP:

Narcotics result in a depression of the respiratory rate and minute ventilation accompanied by an increase in the tidal volume. The result is a slow deep respiratory pattern. The extent of respiratory depression is dose related and reversible with the narcotic antagonist naloxone. An increase in minute ventilation normally corrects any increase in arterial carbon dioxide tension. Narcotics depress this response and elevated levels of $PaCO_2$ may accompany the administration of narcotics.

CVS:

Opioids have little to no myocardial depressant effects even when administered in high doses. Supplementation with either nitrous oxide or benzodiazepines may depress cardiac output. Narcotics decrease systemic vascular resistance (SVR) by either decreasing sympathetic outflow or, in the case of morphine and meperidine, by direct release of histamine. Morphine and meperidine's tendency to release histamine produces vasodilation with a fall in both the blood pressure and SVR. Synthetic opioids, such as fentanyl and its related congeners, are less likely to release histamine. Opioids produce bradycardia by stimulating the vagal nucleus in the brainstem. Meperidine, unlike other narcotics, does not produce bradycardia and may cause significant cardiac depression due to its direct negative ionotropic activity.

GI/GU:

Narcotics slow gastrointestinal mobility and may result in constipation or postoperative ileus. All narcotics increase biliary tract tone and may precipitate biliary colic in patients with cholelithiasis. By increasing the tone of the bladder sphincter, opioids may precipitate postoperative urinary retention. Other, less common, side effects of opioids includes anaphylactic reactions, bronchospasm, chest wall rigidity, and puritis.

Fentanyl, sufentanil, and alfentanil are the most common narcotic agents used during induction and maintenance of anaesthesia. This is due to their rapid onset, and predictable duration of action.

Morphine may be used in the perioperative period to provide long lasting analgesia. It should be administered slowly at a rate not exceeding 5 mg per minute to avoid excessive histamine release.

Meperidine is less commonly used for induction and maintenance of anaesthesia because of its negative ionotropic activity. Hallucinations and nausea are

	Potency Ratio	Analgesic Dose	Low Dose	Moderate Dose	High Dose
Morphine	1	10 mg	0.05 - 0.2 mg/kg	0.2 - 0.3 mg/kg	1 - 2 mg/kg
Meperidine	0.1	100 mg	0.5 - 2.0 mg/kg	2 - 3 mg/kg	---------
Fentanyl	100	100 mcg	0.5 - 3 mcg/kg	3 - 10 mcg/kg	50 - 100 mcg/kg
Sufentanil	500 - 1000	10 -20 mcg	0.1 - 0.2 mcg/kg	0.2 - 1.0 mcg/kg	10 - 30 mcg/kg
Alfentanil	10 - 20	500 -1000 mcg	10 - 20 mcg/kg	10 - 100 mcg/kg	---------

Table 14.1: Comparison of common intraoperative narcotic agonist potencies and doses.
The **'low dose'** schedule represents typical doses administered in divided increments intravenously for perioperative analgesia with inhalational agents when extubation is planned at the end of the procedure.
The **'moderate dose'** schedule represents opioid doses used in combination with a nitrous oxide - relaxant technique, when extubation of the patient is planned within the next four hours.
The **'high dose'** technique is used to induce anaesthesia in patients for whom prolonged postoperative ventilation is planned.

more common with meperidine than with morphine. Normeperidine is an active metabolite of meperidine, which has only half of meperidine's analgesic activity. Normeperidine may cause CNS excitation. In patients receiving large amounts of meperidine for prolonged periods of time, or in patients with renal insufficiency, normeperidine levels may rise significantly and seizure activity may result.

Fentanyl is much more potent than morphine, and because of its high lipid solubility, it has a rapid onset in action. Fentanyl's short duration of action is due to its redistribution from the CNS to other tissue sites in the body.

Sufentanil is the most potent narcotic that is in clinical use today. It has a much smaller volume of distribution than fentanyl, and is ideally suited for intravenous infusion techniques during longer procedures. Infusion rates of 0.1 to 0.5 mcg/kg/hr are appropriate for anaesthesia with an inhalational anaesthetic agent (balanced anaesthesia).

Alfentanil has a rapid onset and rapid recovery and is ideally suited for short procedures requiring intense analgesia.

It has a small volume of distribution and does not accumulate in significant amounts in the body. An intravenous loading dose of 15 - 30 mcg/kg i.v. may be followed with an intravenous infusion rate of 0.25 to 1.5 mcg/kg/min to maintain analgesic plasma levels. Intravenous intermittent bolus doses of 5 - 10 mcg/kg iv may be used to respond to varying intensities of surgical stimulation, while the infusion rate is adjusted. Discontinuation of the infusion 15 - 20 minutes prior to the end of the surgical procedure permits rapid patient awakening for extubation.

Remifentanil:

Remifentanil is the newest addition to our clinically available opioids. It is classified as an ultra-short acting opioid agonist, and has both a rapid onset and peak effect. Adverse side effects such as hypotension, bradycardia, muscle rigidity, and respiratory depression or arrest, may be more pronounced with remifentanil compared to other opioids because of it's rapid onset of action. These side effects are dose and rate of administration dependant and can be reversed with naloxone.

Remifentanil should only be administered by persons specifically trained in the use of anesthestic drugs, and in the recognition and management of it's adverse effects. Immediate measures including the ability to establish and maintain a patent airway and institute controlled ventilation and cardio-respiratory resuscitation must be available when administering remifentanil.

With the exception of using a single 1 mcg/kg bolus intravenous injection during induction of general anesthesia, intravenous bolus administration of remifentanil should only be used in intubated patients during general anesthesia. Remifentanil is ideally suited for administration with an intravenous infusion pump. Infusion doses of 0.1 - 2 ug/kg/min with supplemental bolus doses of 0.5 - 1 ug/kg are recommended during general anesthesia with 66% nitrous oxide in healthy adults.

The rapid offset in action means that within 5 - 10 minutes after stopping an infusion there will be no residual analgesic activity. Patients who are anticipated to have postoperative pain, must have other measures (local anesthesia, NSAID's, long acting opioid administration, etc.), instituted to avoid sudden pain after discontinuing a remifentanil infusion.

Narcotic Antagonists*:
Naloxone (Narcan®) is a pure narcotic antagonist, which competes with opioids at the mu, delta, kappa and sigma receptors. Naloxone is supplied in ampules of 0.02 mg/ml, 0.4 mg/ml, and 1 mg/ml. The 0.4 mg/ml and 1 mg/ml ampules should be diluted with saline to provide a concentration of 0.04 to 0.05 mg/ml for ease of administration.

Naloxone reaches its peak effect within 1 - 2 minutes of intravenous administration, and has a duration of 30 to 60 minutes. Perioperative surgical patients, with evidence of excessive sedation or respiratory depression secondary to opioids, may be given small incremental doses of naloxone of 40 mcg Sudden reversal of the analgesic effects of opioids, however, may result if high doses of naloxone are given. The subsequent abrupt return of pain can result in hypertension, tachycardia, pulmonary edema, ventricular dysrhythmias, and cardiac arrest. Continuous infusions of 3 to 10 mcg/kg/hr of naloxone may be required if sedation or respiratory depression recur.

References:

1. Bailey PL, Stanley. Narcotic intravenous anesthetics. In: Anesthesia. Third edition. Miller RD., ed. Churchill Livingstone Inc. 1990.

2. Hickle RS. Administration of general anesthesia. In: Clinical anaesthesia procedures of the Massachusetts General Hospital. Third edition. Firestone LL, Lebowitz PW, Cook CE., ed. Little, Brown and Company 1988.

3. Barash PG, Cullen BF, Stoelting RK. Opioids. In: Clinical anesthesia. Second edition. JB Lippincott Co., 1993.

Notes:

Notes:

CHAPTER 15

Local and Regional Anaesthesia

Ann Lui M.D., FRCPC

INTRODUCTION

Local and regional anaesthesia plays an important role in modern anaesthetic management. This form of anaesthesia may be used as an alternative to general anaesthesia, or may be used in combination with general anaesthesia in the hope of reducing the severity of the perioperative surgical stress response. While numerous local anaesthetics (LA) are available for use by the clinician, this chapter will focus on three commonly used LA's; Lidocaine, bupivicaine, and chlorprocaine. These three agents illustrate differences in the classification, potency and duration of local anaesthetics. Understanding these agents provides a basis for understanding other local anaesthetic agents that you may use in the future.

LOCAL ANAESTHETICS

Over the next two clinical years you are likely to encounter and use local anaesthetics in many clinical settings. Minor procedures in the emergency room, topical application for eye examination, and local infiltration for diagnostic and therapeutic procedures, are a few common uses of local anaesthetic agents.

Local anaesthetics are drugs that revers-

ibly block impulse conduction in nerve fibers. The molecular structure of most local anaesthetics consists of an aromatic group linked to a hydrophillic amine by either an amide link (amino amides) or an ester link (amino esters). Esters are hydrolysed in the blood by plasma cholinesterase with the formation of paraaminobenzoic acid, a metabolite to which some patients are

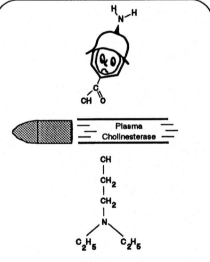

Figure 15.1: Hydrolysis of an ester local anaesthetic by plasma cholinesterase. Amide local anaesthetics undergo metabolism in the liver. Adapted with permission from Tucker, GT. Biotransformation and toxicity of local anaesthetics. Acta Anaesthesiol. Beig., [Supp.];123,1975.

allergic. Unlike ester local anaesthetics, amides are metabolized in the liver and are rarely associated with allergic reactions.

Mechanism of Action*

The mechanism of action of local anaesthetics is not fully understood but most likely involves a dynamic interaction with the sodium channel on the axoplasmic (inner surface) of the nerve membrane.

The nerve cell relies on concentration gradients of ions across its membranes, and selective permeation of ions through its membranes as a basis for maintaining an electrical potential and generating an electrical impulse. The generation of nerve impulses is dependent on the flow of specific ionic currents through channels that span the nerve membrane.

The nerve membrane consists of a fluid lipid bilayer interspersed with protein globules. Local anaesthetics act by passing through the nerve membrane to attach or block the sodium conducting ion channels thereby inhibiting impulse generation.

We will now discuss factors that affect how fast the local anaesthetic acts (onset), how well it blocks impulse generation (potency), and how long it will last (duration).

Agents with a high lipid solubility will penetrate the nerve membrane easily. Hence very lipid soluble agents will move in easily and will appear to be more potent as an anaesthetic. Having penetrated the nerve membrane, LA's that bind strongly to the membranes protein globules will inhibit sodium flux across the nerve membrane for a long period of time. Clinically, we observe a long duration of action when the protein binding of a LA is strong.

The onset of action of the LA is primarily influenced by its pKa. The pKa can be thought of as the pH at which 50% of the LA is in the charged cationic form (BH^+) and 50% is in the uncharged (B) base form.
($BH^+ \rightleftharpoons B + H^+$)

When a local anaesthetic is injected into tissues, it establishes an equilibrium between its two forms (BH^+, and B) which depends on the local pH. In order for the LA to move through the tissues and nerve sheath, it must be in its uncharged base form. Hence, the lower the pKa the higher the concentration of base form and the faster the onset of action. In humans, the starting base form is almost always less than 50% since pKa's are in the range of 7.5 to 8.9 and tissue pH is normally 7.4. Conversely, if you are injecting a local anaesthetic into an infected area with a low pH, the local anaesthetic is ineffective because most of the LA will be in the charged form and unable to penetrate the nerve membrane.

In summary:

Lipid solubility influences potency.
Protein binding influences duration.
And Pka influences onset of action.

Many local anaesthetics have been synthesized since the initial use of the naturally occurring cocaine for ophthalmic procedures. Still a search for the "ideal" drug with the lowest toxicity and best clinical profile continues. The clinical properties that are important include potency, onset of action and duration of action. Table 15.1 lists some of the commonly used local anaesthetics and their clinical properties. Sensory nerves, motor nerves, and autonomic nerves may all be blocked to varying degrees by local anaesthetics.

Bupivicaine has the ability to produce a **differential nerve blockade** when used in dilute concentrations. This form of blockade is especially advantageous in obstetrical patients requiring pain man-agement for labour and delivery. Such a block can provide excellent pain control (sensory nerve block), yet it still allows the patient to move and push during labour (minimal motor nerve blockade). Hence, bupivicaine's ability to provide a differential nerve blockade together with its relatively long duration of action makes it a common choice for epidural pain management in the obstetrical patient.

Lidocaine provides a faster onset (about 10 minutes) but shorter duration (about 1 - 2 hours), as compared with bupivicaine, which has an onset time of up to 30 minutes and a duration of 2 or more hours. Memorizing the relative potencies of the drugs is generally not necessary

	Chlorprocaine	Lidocaine	Bupivicaine
Type	Ester*	Amide*	Amide*
Potency	Low*	Intermediate*	High*
Duration	15 - 30 minutes*	1 - 2 hours*	3 - 8 hours*
Onset	Fast	Fast	Intermediate
Use*	Infiltration Nerve Blocks Epidural	Infiltration Nerve Blocks Epidural Spinal	Infiltration Nerve Blocks Epidural Spinal
Maximum Dose (with epi.)	11 mg/kg (14mg/kg)** 770 mg/ 70 kg 25 ml of 3 %	4 mg/kg (7 mg/kg)** 280 mg / 70 kg 28 ml of 1 %	2.5 mg/kg (3 mg/kg)** 175 mg / 70 kg 35 ml of 0.5 %
Usual Conc.^{n}	1 - 2 % 3 % (Epidural)	0.5 - 2 % 2 % (Epidural) 5 % (Spinal)	0.25 - 0.5 % 0.1 - 0.5 % (Epidural) 0.5 - 0.75 % (Spinal)

Table 15.1: Properties of three commonly used local anaesthetics with the manufacturer's recommended maximum dose for single injection. The maximum dose may be increased by the addition of a vasoconstrictor such as epinephrine. The maximum recommended doses with epinephrine are reported in brackets.

** *Must Know*   * *Should Know*   *Page 115*

as the more potent anaesthetic agents are commercially supplied in lower concentrations (eg. 0.5% bupivicaine with a potency of 8, versus 2% lidocaine with a relative potency of 2).

Toxicity of Local Anaesthetics

How safe are local anaesthetics? We can distinguish the toxic effects of these agents according to their local and systemic effects.

Local toxicities of these agents include direct injury to nervous tissue (neurotoxicity), and direct injury to muscle tissue (myotoxicity). The use of preservatives in the local anaesthetic solution (eg. para-aminobenzoic acid), and the use of a vasoconstrictor such as epinephrine may increase a LA's potential neuro- and myo- toxicities. Direct injection of a LA into a nerve will result in immediate severe pain and will result in pathologic damage to the nerve. If excruciating pain is experienced on injection of a local anaesthetic near a nerve, the injection should be immediately stopped and the needle repositioned. Injection of LA's into muscles may result in histological changes in the tissues. These are, however, generally transient, reversible and clinically insignificant.

Systemic toxicities involve the central nervous system, the cardiovascular system, and the respiratory system. Figure 15.2 shows the positive relationship between symptoms of systemic toxicity and increasing plasma levels of lidocaine. Systemic complications are more likely to occur when a large dose of local anaesthetic is rapidly injected into, or near blood vessels. To avoid these systemic side effects, inject slowly, aspirate to check for intravascular entry, consider adding a vasoconstrictor like epinephrine, to retard vascular absorption, and do not exceed the maximum recommended dosage.

Most clinicians have difficulty recalling the maximum safe dose when administering a local anaesthetic. Fortunately, the local anaesthetics are commercially prepared such that the bottle with the highest concentration of drug contains less than the maximum dosage for the average 70 kg adult. For example lidocaine's highest concentration for regional anaesthesia is 2% (20 mg/mL). One vial's volume of 20 mL (total 400 mg) is within the limit of the maximum dosage, if epinephrine is present in the lidocaine. Generally, if the volume of the local anaesthetic with epinephrine is restricted to a maximum of one bottle (20 mL) per adult patient, the clinician will remain within the safe limit for the total allowable dose. The solution can be diluted (with preservative free saline) if a greater volume of local anaesthetic is required.

The potential for systemic toxicity of local anaesthetics increases with the concentration of the local anaesthetic in the blood. Absorption of LA's in the blood can be decreased by the addition of a vasoconstrictor such as epinephrine or phenylephrine. Typical concentrations of epinephrine that are used are 1:100,00 to 1:200:000. A 1:200,000 concentration of epinephrine has 5 mcg/mL of epinephrine, or 0.1 mL of

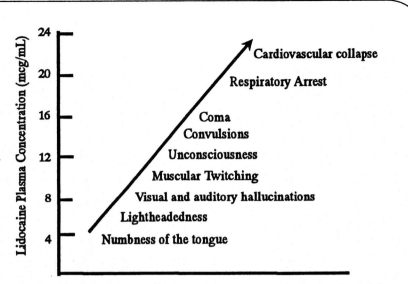

Figure 15.2: Relationship of signs and symptoms of local anaesthetic toxicity to plasma concentrations of lidocaine. With permission from Covino B.G., Clinical pharmacology of local anaesthetics. In Neural Blockade. Cousins MJ, Bridenbaugh (Eds.) 2nd edition J.B. Lippincott 1980.

epinephrine (1 mg/mL concentration) added to 20 mL of LA.

The uptake of local anaesthetics into the blood will be accelerated if injected in the proximity of major blood vessels (fig. 15.3). Intercostal nerve blocks result in the highest peak local anaesthetic blood concentrations, whereas infiltrative injection achieves the lowest peak serum levels, provided direct intravascular injection is avoided.

The potential for systemic toxicity is very real. High concentrations of LA in the blood may result in a spectrum of symptoms reflecting an initial excitation of the CNS followed by CNS, respiratory, and cardiovascular depression. In severe cases, this may be observed as a sudden loss of consciousness, respiratory arrest, or cardiovascular arrest. When the clinician administers a large dose of a local anaesthetic, the patient should be closely monitored by main-

Intercostal Nerve Block
↓
Epidural Anaesthesia
↓
Femoral/Brachial Plexus Block
↓
Peripheral Nerve Block
↓
Local Infiltration

Fig. 15.3: Regional blocks in decreasing order of systemic absorption and the potential for systemic toxic reactions.

Table 15.2:	Treatment of Acute Local Anaesthetic Toxicity**
Ensure a clear airway.	Utilize manoeuvres such as suctioning, chin lift, jaw thrust, insertion of oral and nasal airways, and positioning the patient in the lateral decubitus position.
Ensure adequate ventilation.	Manually assist or control the patient's breathing using an Ambu bag and mask unit. Avoid respiratory acidosis secondary to hypoventilation, as this will increase the local anaesthetic uptake and toxicity. If unable to control ventilation by mask, consider intubation (may require succinylcholine 1 mg/kg iv).
Provide supplemental oxygen.	Ensure the patient is receiving supplemental oxygen. Set the ambu bag oxygen flow at 8 to 10 l/min.
Assess the heart rate and rhythm, apply monitors.	Treat bradycardia with atropine. Initial dose of 1 mg iv., followed by 0.5 mg iv every 5 mins. to a max. of 3 mg. Use epinephrine as per ACLS guidelines for profound cardiovascular collapse. Consider early electrical cardioversion for arrhythmias.
Assess the blood pressure and perfusion (determine responsiveness).	If the patient is hypotensive, place them in the trendelenburg position. Administer an initial fluid bolus of 500 to 1000 ml of saline or ringer's lactate. Support blood pressure with ephedrine 5 - 10 mg, or phenylephrine 50 mcg iv prn every 2 - 3 minutes.
Stop seizures.	Protect the patient from physical injury during a seizure. Consider administering 5 - 10 mg of diazepam iv, or 50 mg of sodium thiopental to stop the seizure.

taining verbal contact, as well as by continuous ECG monitoring, pulse oximetry, and blood pressure readings.

Management of CNS, respiratory, and cardiovascular toxicity** begins with the ABCs (airway, breathing, and circulation) followed by the ACLS recommendations for resuscitation. The only deviation in the algorithm is the avoidance of the use of Class Ia and Ib antiarrhythmics such as procainamide, quinidine, and lidocaine. These agents are themselves local anaesthetics. Hence, any local anaesthetic induced arrhythmia will be exacerbated by their administration. In the case of LA toxicity and life threatening arrhythmias, bretylium is the agent of choice. Epinephrine can be used if indicated, according to the ACLS guidelines.

REGIONAL ANAESTHESIA

Many studies have examined the benefits of regional over general anaesthesia. Still, there is continuing controversy regarding the best type of anaesthetic.

Perhaps, *what type of anaesthetic* is chosen may not be as important as how well the anaesthetist administers it.

Table 15.3: Reported Benefits of Regional Anaesthesia	
Benefits	**Importance**
► Decreased perioperative nausea and emesis	Decreased hospital stay, improved patient satisfaction
► Reduced perioperative blood loss	Orthopaedic surgery for total hip arthroplasty, prostatic surgery.
► Reduced perioperative stress indicators	Decreased catecholamines
► Ability to monitor CNS status during the procedure	Detection of myocardial ischemia, monitoring CNS status during prostatic surgery (TURP syndrome) and carotid artery surgery
► Improved vascular perfusion	Improved perioperative patency of vascular grafts (eg. Femoral - popliteal vascular graft)
► Reduced deep vein thrombosis	Reduced incidence of pulmonary embolism
► Reduced perioperative pulmonary complications	Reduced incidence of atelectasis, pneumonia
► Reduced perioperative analgesic requirements (pre-emptive analgesia)	Decreased costs and side effects of other anaesthetic agents

Table 15.3 summarizes some of the benefits of regional anaesthesia.

It is convenient to distinguish how local anaesthetics can be administered. The various routes of administration include: topical anaesthesia, infiltrative anaesthesia, intravenous regional anaesthesia, peripheral neural blockade, and central neural blockade.

Topical Anaesthesia

There are various preparations of local anaesthetics available for topical use. They must be able to penetrate the surface (either mucous membrane or skin). Cocaine 4% or 10% is often used for anaesthetizing nasal mucosa. As this is the only local anaesthetic that inhibits noradrenaline uptake resulting in its catecholamine effects it has vasoconstricting properties that "shrink" the mucosa and effect some hemostasis during procedures. Lidocaine 2% jelly is used for intra urethral procedures and catheter insertion.

In Canada, EMLA (a 1:1 eutectic mixture of 25 mg lidocaine and 25 mg prilocaine per gram of cream) is available in 5g or 30g tubes for application on the skin. The cream must be applied under an occlusive dressing (e.g., tegaderm®) for more than 60 minutes to achieve dermal analgesia to a depth of 3mm. About 5 to 10% of the drug is absorbed systemically. EMLA is an effective topical anaesthetic for intravenous catheter insertion, blood sampling and minor skin surgery (e.g., laser treatment, wart removal). This preparation is not recommended for use on mucous membranes.

Infiltrative Anaesthesia

Also referred to as local infiltration, this technique involves injection of local anaesthetic intradermally, subcutaneously or in the tissue within the vicinity of the area of surgery. When large areas are involved, avoid using more than one bottle of local anaesthetic. Instead, one may dilute the solution to give the volume required to cover the area.

Intravenous Regional Anaesthesia "Bier Block"

This technique is very useful for anaesthetizing the distal arm or leg for procedures of 1 hour or less. ECG, BP, and oximetry monitors are applied prior to performing the block. An intravenous is secured in the non-operative extremity for prn drug administration and emergency use. A second small intravenous is inserted in the distal extremity for injection of the LA. A tourniquet is applied to the limb and tested for its ability to abolish the extremities pulse by maintaining a pressure of 100 mm Hg above the systolic BP. The limb is elevated, wrapped with an elastic bandage (esmarch) to ex-

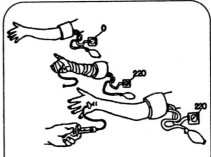

Figure 15.4: Intravenous regional anaesthesia commonly referred to as a 'Bier Block'. With permission from Covino BG., Lambert DH. In: Anesthesiology principles and procedures. Lui PL. (ed.) JB Lippincott Co. 1992.

anguinate the limb, and the tourniquet is inflated. The esmarch bandage is removed, loss of arterial pulse confirmed, and a solution of 0.25 - 0.5% lidocaine plain (without preservative) is slowly injected in the operative limb's iv, (max. 3 mg/kg). The local anaesthetic diffuses from the venous vascular bed into the tissues to provide operative anaesthesia within 5 minutes. Care must be taken to ensure proper function of the tourniquet if success is to be achieved and a sudden iv infusion of lidocaine is to be avoided. A minimum of 20 minutes tourniquet time is needed to allow adequate tissue uptake of the local anaesthetic to avoid toxic reactions on deflation of the tourniquet. The technique is illustrated in figure 15.4.

Peripheral Nerve Blockade

Local anaesthetics can be deposited close to individual nerves (e.g., the ulnar nerve, median nerve, or femoral nerve), or to the nerve plexus (e.g., brachial plexus and lumbosacral plexus). A thorough knowledge of the anatomy of the peripheral nervous system is important to locate the site of injection as well as to determine whether the technique will provide adequate anaesthesia for the surgical site. There are many well illustrated texts and workshops that describe each nerve or plexus block that can be used as a guide. The most devastating complication of peripheral nerve blockade is nerve injury which can be minimized if two cardinal rules* are practiced:

1. **Avoid intraneural injection.**
2. **Avoid neurotoxic agents.**

An intraneural injection can be detected when patients complain of excruciating pain in the distribution of the affected nerve at the start of the injection. Stop and withdraw the needle if this occurs. Intraneural injection of less than 0.5 ml of solution can raise intraneural pressures to ischemic levels resulting in permanent damage. Use an atraumatic needle; one specifically designed for nerve blockade, the nerve tends to "roll off" the blunt end of these needles, rather than being impaled.

Most preservatives contained in the local anaesthetic solutions have the potential to be neurotoxic. All solutions selected for peripheral nerve block (including the normal saline used for diluting the solutions) should, therefore, be **free of preservatives** as indicated on the bottle.

Central Neural Blockade

Central neural blockade refers to either epidural or spinal anaesthesia. Epidural anaesthesia involves injecting drugs into the epidural space, which lies between the ligamentum flavum and the dura mater, exterior to the spinal fluid. Spinal anaesthesia involves passing a needle through the epidural space, through the dura and into the CSF (intrathecal) space, see figure 15.5 and 15.6.

In spinal anaesthesia, the local anaesthetic is injected into the subarachnoid

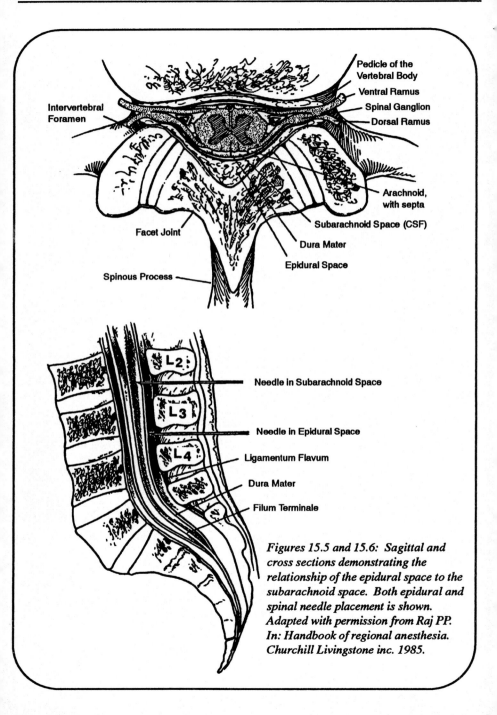

Figures 15.5 and 15.6: Sagittal and
cross sections demonstrating the
relationship of the epidural space to the
subarachnoid space. Both epidural and
spinal needle placement is shown.
Adapted with permission from Raj PP.
In: Handbook of regional anesthesia.
Churchill Livingstone inc. 1985.

space (CSF containing space), where it is in direct contact with the "bare" nerve roots. By contrast, local anaesthetics administered in the epidural space must pass through the myelin sheaths covering the nerve roots. The dura acts as a barrier to epidural LA's moving into the CSF space. Local anaesthetics that contact the nerves directly, as in spinal anaesthesia, produce a very rapid and intense nerve block. By contrast, epidural anaesthesia has a slower onset because the nerves are, in a sense insulated, and it produces a less intense block. Epidural anaesthesia typically requires 5 - 10 times the amount of LA that would be used for spinal anaesthesia.

Continuous infusions of local anaesthetics and opioids into the epidural space can be used intraoperatively and continued postoperatively. Both spinal and epidural anaesthesia affect motor, sensory and sympathetic nerves in the neural axis. Nerve blockade of the sympathetic nervous system results in vasodilation, which in turn decreases venous return, stroke volume and cardiac output. If this produces

Table 15.4: Spinal and Epidural Anaesthesia	
Contraindications*	Complications

Patient refusal
Lack of resuscitative equipment
Lack of knowledge of procedure
Coagulopathy
Previous back surgery (relative)
Raised intracranial pressure
Fixed cardiac output:
  - severe aortic or mitral stenosis
  - IHSS
Pre-existing neurologic disease
  - ALS, Multiple sclerosis
	Inadequate anaesthesia
	Excessive anaesthesia
	  - 'High block' with potential
	    respiratory insufficiency and
	    cardiovascular collapse.
	Sympathetic blockade (hypotension)
	Dural puncture (headache)
	Injury:
	  - muscles, ligaments, bone
	    (back pain)
	  - nerve root or spinal cord
	    (nerve deficit)
	  - epidural vien (epidural hematoma)
	  - anterior spinal artery
	    (nerve deficit)
	Infection:
	  - bone (osteitis)
	  - epidural space (epidural abscess)
	  - CSF (meningitis)
	Inadvertent intravascular injection of
	local anaesthetic: see text re: local
	anaesthetic toxicity.

hypotension, it is first treated with fluid boluses and, if necessary a sympathomimetic drug such as ephedrine (see chapter 22).

Sympathetic blockade of the cardioaccelerator fibres at levels T1 to T4 can result in unopposed vagal effects causing bradycardia, or even asystole. Progressive bradycardia and hypotension under spinal anaesthesia are warning signs that suggest the block may be reaching the cardioaccelerator fibres. A combination of intravenous fluids, atropine, ephedrine, or phenylephrine ought to be used to treat these hemodynamic abnormalities as soon as they are recognized.

Nevertheless, misconceptions and unwarranted concern about complications of epidural and spinal anaesthesia are common in both the lay and medical profession. The risks of a life threatening or debilitating complication occurring after epidural or spinal anaesthesia are probably less than the risks we take when we ride in our car. Table 15.4 lists the contraindications and potential complications of central neural blockade.

The discomfort experienced with the performance of an epidural or spinal block is comparable to that experienced when an intravenous is inserted. If inadequate local anaesthesia is used to perform the block, or if musculoskeletal abnormalities are present, finding the epidural or intrathecal space may be more difficult. In this situation, pain may be experienced from injury to the adjacent muscles, ligaments, bone, nerve roots, or spinal cord.

Injury to the muscles, ligaments, and bone may result in transient discomfort, that can be treated with oral analgesics and rest. An injury to a nerve root or the spinal cord is very rare. The awake patient will experience severe pain if the spinal cord or a nerve root is touched, at which point the clinician should reposition the needle, to avoid permanent injury. As the spinal cord terminates between the 1st and 2nd lumbar vertebral body in adults, insertion of an epidural or spinal needle in the low lumbar region (i.e., L3 - L4) reduces the risk of direct damage to the spinal cord.

Whenever the dura is punctured, there is a risk that the patient will develop a postural headache, referred to as a "dural puncture headache". The dura is intentionally punctured when performing spinal anaesthesia, it may be inadvertently punctured with an epidural needle if the needle is advanced past the epidural space. The chance of a dural puncture headache varies with the size and type of needle used, direction of the bevel, and age of the patient. For instance, young patients who have their dura punctured with a large bore (16 ga. epidural needle) have about a 60% chance of developing a headache. This headache may be quite debilitating and persist for two or more weeks. Sometimes another procedure called an "epidural blood patch" is required to treat this headache.

The risk of an inadvertent dural puncture when an epidural is performed is approximately 1:100 to 1:200 patients. Young patients having a dural puncture for spinal anaesthesia with a small needle (eg. 27 ga. needle) have a 1 - 3 % chance of developing a headache. Elderly patients do not seem to be prone to this complication.

Permanent neurologic damage following central neural blockade is very rare. This can occur if: direct nerve trauma occurs, infection is introduced into the spinal canal, a neurotoxic drug is injected by mistake, or an epidural hematoma develops and compresses the nerve roots. Historically there are reports of paraplegia following the use of epidural or spinal anaesthetics contaminated with neurotoxic chemicals or with bacteria. Despite this, the currently available local anaesthetics are safe when used in the appropriate doses.

Although extra care should be taken when inserting an epidural or spinal anaesthetic in the patient with low back pain, this is not a contraindication to performing the block. Moreover, the incidence of postoperative low back pain in patients who had regional as compared to general anaesthesia is not significantly different. In fact, patients with chronic back pain problems benefit from epidural injections of local anaesthetics and steroids.

Undoubtedly, some risk is associated with any form of anaesthesia. Still the risks of general anaesthesia are greater than those for central neural blockade in some cases. For example, epidural or spinal anaesthesia are preferred to general anaesthesia for caesarean sections. This is because we recognize that the two greatest causes of morbidity and mortality in pregnant patients having a general anaesthetic are aspiration of gastric contents and the failure to intubate, both of which are avoided by using regional anaesthesia.

References:

1. Cousins MJ, Bridenbaugh PO. (ed.) Neural Blockade in Clinical Anesthesia and Management of Pain. Second Edition. JB Lippincott Co.1988.

2. Miller RD. (ed) Anesthesia. Third Edition. Churchill Livingstone Inc. 1990.

Notes:

CHAPTER 16

Acute Pain Management

JOHN PENNING M.D., FRCPC

INTRODUCTION

The last few decades has brought vast improvements in the understanding and management of acute pain. Many new and effective treatment modalities are now available, including patient controlled analgesia (PCA) and administration of neuraxial (epidural or spinal) opioids. Anaesthesiologists are highly knowledgeable in opioid pharmacology, and are experts at spinal and epidural drug delivery. In the 1980's, acute pain services were developed under the direction of the departments of anaesthesiology and nursing, at leading centres throughout the world. We have learned that acute pain management is attainable and that the optimization of acute pain management leads to better patient outcome and shorter hospital stays. Poorly controlled acute pain is causally related to perioperative morbidity and mortality. The investment in acute pain management has been cost effective for both hospitals and society as a whole.

Despite remarkable progress in certain centres in the management of acute pain, intramuscular morphine or meperidine on an as needed (p.r.n.) basis remain the most popular form of acute postoperative pain management at most Canadian hospitals. Even so, specialists in pain management regard intramuscular opioid administration as a technique that provides inferior pain control when compared to other techniques currently available.

This discrepancy between recommended and actual pain management techniques, spurred the American Agency for Health Care Policy and Research Development towards developing clinical practice guidelines for acute pain management. This extensive work involved the review of thousands of articles and consultation with hundreds of leading world experts. The results were published in February 1992 under the title: "Acute Pain Management: Operative or Medical Procedures and Trauma[1]". This well regarded clinical practice guideline promises to set the standard in pain management for 1990's.

We will now proceed with a review of some basic neurophysiology of acute pain. Following this, we shall review the principles of analgesia therapy with PCA, neuraxial opioids and non steroidal anti-inflammatory drugs (NSAIDs).

NOCICEPTION*:

Nociception refers to the detection, transduction and transmission of noxious stimuli. Substances generated from thermal, mechanical or chemical tissue damage, activate free nerve endings, which we refer to as nociceptors. These peripheral afferent neurons have their cell body located in the dorsal root ganglion and send axonal projections into the dorsal horn and other areas of the spinal cord (figure 16.1). Synapses occur with a second order afferent neuron, as well as with regulatory interneurons. In addition, synapses occur with the cell bodies of the sympathetic nervous system and ventral motor nuclei, either directly or through the internuncial neurons. These circuits are important for understanding the reflex sympathetic and motor responses that result from segmental afferent nociceptive input to the spinal cord.

The cell body of the second order neuron lies in the dorsal horn. Axonal projections of this neuron cross to the contralateral hemisphere of the spinal cord and ascend to the level of the thalamus. Along the way, this neuron divides and sends axonal branches that synapse in the regions of the reticular formation, nucleus raphe magnus, periaqueductal gray, and other areas of the brain stem. In the thalamus, the second order neuron synapses with a third order afferent neuron, which sends axonal projections into the sensory cortex.

CLINICAL RELEVANCE** OF ACUTE PAIN PATHOPHYSIOLOGY:

A goal of all health care providers should be to provide optimal acute pain management. Indeed, some of the morbidity and mortality that patients experience after trauma or major surgery may be the final result of the pathological disturbances that are initiated by severe and poorly controlled acute pain.

Patients with large chest wall or abdominal incisions, who do not receive adequate acute pain control, experience significant chest, abdominal and diaphragmatic muscle splinting that limits their ability to breathe deeply and to cough. This impairs their ability to clear airway secretions. The patient is rendered prone to atelectasis (collapse of segmental lung regions), which increases the risk of hypoxemia and pneumonia. This muscle splinting is a reflex response to acute pain stimuli at the level of the spinal cord. It can be prevented or alleviated by appropriate analgesic therapy.

The barrage of nociceptive stimuli reaching the spinal cord also initiates spinally and supra-spinally mediated reflex increases in sympathetic tone. This results in hypertension, tachycardia, increased contractility and an increase in the work demanded of the heart. If this occurs in a setting of decreased oxygen supply, due to blood loss and decreased lung efficiency, myocardial ischemia, congestive heart failure and myocardial infarction may result.

The increased sympathetic tone during acute pain also increases intestinal secretions, slows gut motility, and increases smooth muscle tone. These changes may lead to gastric stasis with nausea, vomiting, ileus and urinary retention.

Poorly controlled acute pain plays a significant role in initiating and maintaining the *stress-response* associated with the trauma of major surgery. This response includes the development of a *hyper-coagulable* state, which can lead to deep vein thrombosis, pulmonary

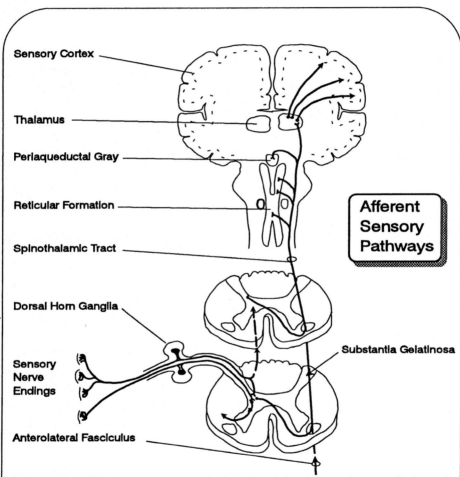

Figure 16.1 Afferent sensory pathways for detection and transmission of nociceptive impulses. Modified with permission from Lubenow TR, McCarthy RJ, Ivankovich AD: Management of acute postoperative pain. In Barash PG, Cullen BF, Stoelting RK (eds): Clinical Anesthesia, 2nd ed. Philadelphia: JB Lippincott, 1992.

embolism and myocardial infarction in the postoperative period. Further changes associated with the stress response to trauma include decreased immunocompetence, hyper-metabolism and mobilization of energy stores. These responses explain the tendency toward hyperglycemia and large net protein losses that sometimes delay wound healing.

MODULATION OF NOCICEPTION:

Afferent neurons transmit information from peripheral pain receptors to the CNS. Efferent neurons descend from the brainstem to the dorsal horn to decrease incoming nociceptive information.

The peripheral and central components of the nervous system that serve to detect, transduce and transmit nociceptive signals are subject to control from higher centres within the CNS. This serves in a *negative feed-back fashion* to limit the amount of afferent nociceptive stimulation that can be perceived as pain. Modulation can occur either in the periphery or at any point where synaptic transmission occurs. Anatomically, the most important site where modulation occurs is in the outer layers of the dorsal horn, named the substantia gelatinosa. This is where the synapse between the primary afferent sensory neuron and the secondary afferent sensory neuron occurs.

Propagation of a sensory impulse from the primary to the secondary sensory neuron depends on the release of an adequate amount of neurotransmitter capable of diffusing across the synapse, binding to the specific synaptic receptors and causing depolarization of the secondary neuron. Substance "P" is a neuropeptide that acts as a neurotransmitter in this fashion. There are several neurotransmitter substances released by modulatory neurons within the substantia gelatinosa that dampen transmission either by impairing the release of the neurotransmitter (such as substance "P") or by rendering the neuron's post-junctional membrane more difficult to depolarize.

Examples of such modulatory neurotransmitters include: endorphins and enkephalins, norepinephrine, serotonin, and gamma amino butyric acid. Pain killers, such as the opioid narcotics (morphine, meperidine), mimic the action of the body's own pain killers (endorphins, enkephalins) by dampening the afferent pain signals being transmitted to the CNS.

There are also occasions when signals are amplified rather than dampened. Although the mechanisms involved are complex, the important principle is that the system is not static. It **does not** function like a *hard wired* electrical circuit board. The system is dynamic and subject to change in how the nociceptive signals are handled. Investigators have coined the term *neuronal plasticity*, to underscore this principle.

OPIOIDS:

This highly effective class of analgesics operates at several levels in the nervous system. They directly dampen the transmission of nociception across the synapse between primary and secondary nociceptive afferent neurons in the dorsal horn by binding to pre-synaptic, post-synaptic or interneuron opioid receptors within the substantia gelatinosa of the dorsal horn.

They activate descending efferent modulatory pathways, resulting in the release of inhibitory neurotransmitters such as noradrenaline, serotonin and GABA. These efferent modulatory neurons originate in the brain stem (i.e., peri-aqueductal grey) and travel down the spinal cord in the dorsolateral fasciculus to terminate in the dorsal horn (figure 16.3).

Opioids inhibit the inflammatory response in the periphery and decrease hyperalgesia. Opioids also affect mood and anxiety by their activity at opioid receptors in the limbic regions of the brain. This helps alleviate the affective component of the perceived pain.

Oral analgesics are generally limited for use in patients with mild postoperative pain. Moderate to severe acute postoperative pain is poorly controlled with oral analgesics alone. This is due to their prolonged time to reach peak effect, lack of flexibility in titration, and dependence on a functional GI tract.

INTRAMUSCULAR OPIOID ADMINISTRATION: LIMITATIONS DUE TO PHARMACOLOGIC PRINCIPLES

Inadequate analgesia: The intermittent administration of intramuscular (i.m.) opioids, every three to four hours, results in a cyclical pattern of peaks and troughs in the serum opioid levels. There is a significant time delay between the i.m. administration and the attainment of adequate pain relief due to the slow and variable rate of drug absorption from the i.m. depot. Austin et al. found that the average peak serum level after 100 mg of meperidine (Demerol®) occurred 44 minutes after i.m. administration (range 15 - 110 minutes). They also noted a five fold variability in the maximum concentration attained and a three fold variability in the minimum effective serum concentration for meperidine. This 3 to 4 fold inter-patient variability in the minimum effective drug concentration has also been observed for other opioids. Hence after i.m. opioid injections, the peak concentrations attained are often sub therapeutic.

Those patients who do have adequate analgesia at peak levels are still subject to sub-therapeutic levels during the trough portions of the serum opioid cycle, which accounts for 30 - 50% of the time. This is especially true in the early post-operative period when the pain is the most intense and the drug levels fall quickly due to a rapid redistribution within the patient's central compartment.

High incidence of side effects:
When opioids are administered intermittently (every 3 to 4 hours) by i.m. injection, the therapeutic window during which the effective concentration of the drug is reached, may last only a fraction of the time between injections. This

reflects the large variability among patients in the maximum drug level reached in the blood after i.m. injections, and the large variability in the effective drug concentration among patients (see figure 16.4). The conse-

quence of having too little drug is pain with all of its adverse sequelae. The side effects of too much opioid in the system are sedation, respiratory depression, puritis, and an increased incidence of nausea and vomiting.

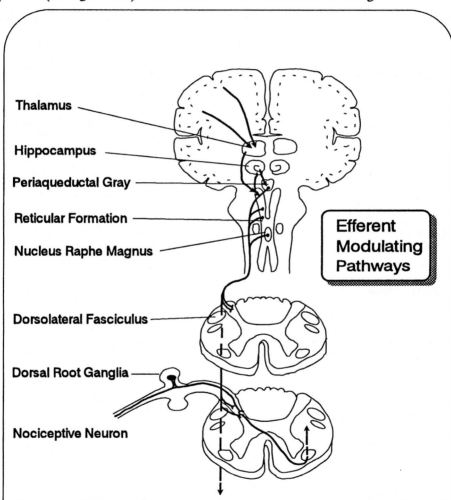

Thalamus

Hippocampus

Periaqueductal Gray

Reticular Formation

Nucleus Raphe Magnus

Efferent Modulating Pathways

Dorsolateral Fasciculus

Dorsal Root Ganglia

Nociceptive Neuron

Figure 16.2 Efferent pathways involved in nociceptive regulation. Modified with permission from Lubenow TR, McCarthy RJ, Ivankovich AD: Management of acute postoperative pain. In Barash PG, Cullen BF, Stoelting RK (eds): Clinical Anesthesia, 2nd ed. Philadelphia: JB Lippincott, 1992:1548.

OPIOIDS BY CONTINUOUS INFUSION:

This approach generally provides post-operative analgesia that is superior to prn i.m. injections. It has the advantage of being simple and avoids repeated and painful i.m. injections. Unfortunately, as with i.m. opioids, this modality lacks sufficient flexibility. The maximum rate of drug delivery *allowable* is often

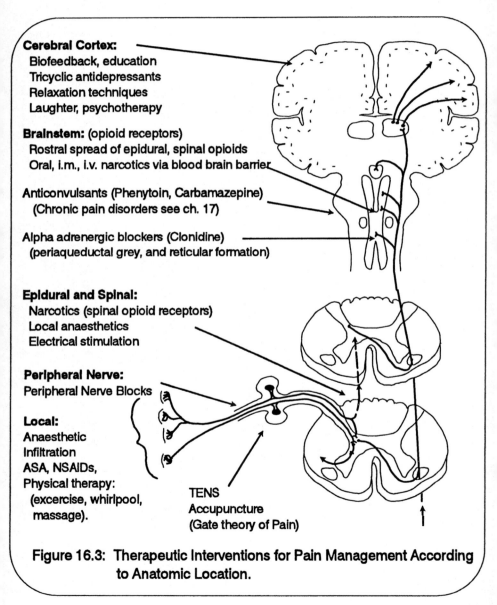

Cerebral Cortex:
Biofeedback, education
Tricyclic antidepressants
Relaxation techniques
Laughter, psychotherapy

Brainstem: (opioid receptors)
Rostral spread of epidural, spinal opioids
Oral, i.m., i.v. narcotics via blood brain barrier

Anticonvulsants (Phenytoin, Carbamazepine)
  (Chronic pain disorders see ch. 17)

Alpha adrenergic blockers (Clonidine)
  (periaqueductal grey, and reticular formation)

Epidural and Spinal:
Narcotics (spinal opioid receptors)
Local anaesthetics
Electrical stimulation

Peripheral Nerve:
Peripheral Nerve Blocks

Local:
Anaesthetic
Infiltration
ASA, NSAIDs,
Physical therapy:
  (excercise, whirlpool,
  massage).

TENS
Accupuncture
(Gate theory of Pain)

Figure 16.3: Therapeutic Interventions for Pain Management According to Anatomic Location.

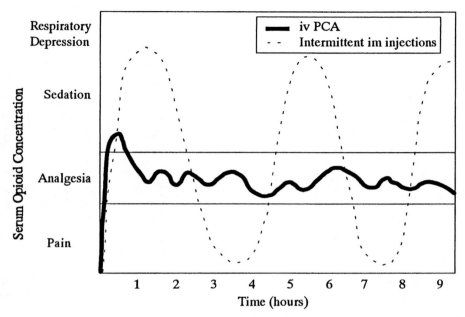

Figure 16.4: Wide fluctuations in serum opioid concentrations are associated with their intermittent intramuscular administration. This results in periods of over-sedation alternating with periods of poor pain control. By contrast, intravenous PCA opioid administration can be rapidly adjusted by the patient. This permits analgesic concentrations of opioids in the serum to be maintained for prolonged periods of time.

insufficient, especially early in the acute post-operative period when the drug may redistribute quickly away from the therapeutic site in the CNS to the peripheral compartment. However, after several hours, the tissues can become *saturated* and the serum drug levels may begin to rise to dangerous levels. This means that closer nursing supervision must be supplied for patients that are on continuous opioid infusions than patients on intravenous patient controlled analgesia (i.v. PCA). Patients in acute pain starting on a continuous infusion of an opioid will require an initial bolus loading dose to quickly achieve analgesic levels. A continuous infusion will then maintain stable plasma levels.

A continuous opioid intravenous infusion is not able to respond to *breakthrough pain* occurring during periods of ambulation, or chest physiotherapy. Adjustment of the infusion rate may take hours to reach the effective analgesic concentration, (typically 4 - 5 times the drugs half life to reach a steady state). By contrast, i.v. PCA plasma levels can be temporarily increased when the patient requests additional doses, allowing the effective concentration to be reached within minutes.

In centres without a PCA service, an alternative may be a low background infusion of narcotic (eg. morphine 0.5 - 2 mg i.v. per hour), with added p.r.n. subcutaneous injections for periods of need (eg. morphine 5 - 7.5 mg s.q. or i.m. q 3 hours). This avoids over sedation with high infusion rates, which is especially important in   patients at night. It is important that infusion rates are decreased as pain levels decline or sedation appears. The time required to achieve analgesia with this technique will be slower than i.v. PCA due to time required for:

1. The patient to signal to the nurse that pain control is inadequate.
2. The nurse to draw up and administer the pain medication.
3. The time it takes for the opioid to be absorbed from the s.c. or i.m. injection site.

I.V. PCA
INTRAVENOUS PATIENT CONTROLLED ANALGESIA

Pharmacological aspects: The direct i.v. administration of an opioid results in a rapid peak in the serum drug level. The time to onset of analgesia depends upon the rate at which the opioid is able to diffuse from plasma to the CNS, where binding to specific analgesia opioid receptors occurs.   The major factor determining the diffusion of the opioid from the plasma to the CNS is the drug's lipid solubility. Table 16.1 lists the opioid analgesia time profiles fol-

lowing a typical PCA bolus of opioid drug.

The rapid onset of analgesia allows the i.v. PCA modality to respond quickly to conditions where *breakthrough pain* may occur (e.g., chest physiotherapy or ambulation). An appropriate bolus dose of i.v. opioid will be smaller than an i.m. dose, but can be given more frequently. An i.m. injection results in lower peak serum levels of drug with a delay in the peak level when compared with an i.v. injection. An i.m. injection also results in a storage depot, which continues to release drug after it has been administered.

The duration of effect after an i.v. bolus of opioid depends upon the rate at which the drug is cleared away from the opioid receptor sites within the CNS. This is determined by the drug's ability to diffuse through neural tissues, a characteristic referred to as lipophilicity. The duration of effect is also determined by the rate at which the drug is cleared from the plasma by redistribution, metabolism, and excretion.

Morphine with its low lipophilicity, diffuses slowly into and out of neural tissue. This results in a slower onset and a longer duration of action when compared with other commonly used opioids. The level of analgesia from morphine does not closely parallel morphine's serum concentration because of a time lag between the concentration at the opioid receptor and in the serum. By contrast, more lipophilic drugs, such as meperidine and fentanyl, diffuse into and out of the CNS quickly and their

| Table 16.1: Time profiles for the clinical effects of i.v. PCA opioids. ||||
Drug	Onset (mins.)	Peak Effect (mins.)	Duration (mins.)
Morphine	3 - 6	20 - 30	40 - 60
Meperidine	2 - 4	8 - 12	20 - 30
Fentanyl	1 - 2	4 - 6	6 - 10
Alfentanil	< 1/2	1 - 2	3 - 5

plasma levels reflect the opioid receptor level concentration and their clinical effect.

In summary, i.v. PCA has the following advantages over i.m. opioid injections for pain control:

1. Rapid onset of analgesia.
2. Eliminates wide fluctuations in plasma opioid concentrations that follow i.m. administration (fewer side effects with better pain control).
3. Accommodates patient variability in opioid dose requirements.
4. Accommodates changes in opioid requirements during the recovery period.
5. Patients benefit psychologically when they have control over pain.
6. Avoids painful i.m. injections.
7. Decreases the risk of accidental needle-stick injury to health care providers.
8. Improves patient-nurse relations. (The patient regards the nurse as a professional who is helping them optimize PCA use, rather than someone who is withholding pain medications).
9. May decrease morbidity and allow for earlier discharge from hospital.

PCA PARAMETERS:

There are five parameters that define PCA therapy:

1. The Loading Dose: This is generally reserved for patients requiring immediate pain medication. Administration of small bolus doses will take too long to achieve the required plasma concentrations because of the lockout interval. A typical loading dose is 0.1 - 0.2 mg/kg for morphine, administered over 10 to 20 minutes. Most postoperative patients will have received narcotics during their procedure and will not require a loading dose when PCA is started after their surgery.

2. The Bolus Dose: This is the amount of opioid delivered to the patient when the patient presses the PCA demand button requesting pain medication. This should be large enough for patients to perceive an analgesic effect, but not so large that the therapeutic window is exceeded (resulting in side effects). For morphine, a typical bolus dose is 1 mg (range 0.5 - 2 mg); for meperidine 10 mg (range 5 - 20 mg).

3. <u>The Lockout Interval:</u> The PCA pump is programmed to deliver another bolus dose only after a specified period of time (called the lockout interval) has elapsed since the last bolus dose. If a patient presses the button before the lockout interval has elapsed, a demand request will be recorded, however, no drug will be delivered. This allows time to elapse for the bolus dose to have an effect (see table 16.1). Typical lockout intervals are 5 to 10 minutes.

4. <u>Continuous Infusion:</u> In addition to giving the patient a bolus of narcotic when requested, a continuous iv infusion can be also be administered (ordered as *PCA + continuous infusion*). Typical infusion rates for morphine (and for meperidine,) are 0.5 - 1.0 mg per hour and 5 - 10 mg per hour. There is debate over the benefits of a continuous infusion with PCA. Proponents of this technique argue that it prevents patients from waking in the night with severe pain because they have not received pain medication for several hours. Still, studies show no clear benefits of a continuous infusion over PCA alone. A continuous infusion places these patients at risk of respiratory depression and other complications of excess opioid use. When used in the early postoperative period, we recommend that the infusion be discontinued (*PCA mode alone*) as soon as the patient's bolus demands decrease to to 2 per four hours.

5. <u>Maximum 4 hour Limit:</u> Like the infusion parameter, this parameter is also not essential, but may be set at the physician's discretion. It provides an extra safeguard against a programming error, which may occur while setting up the PCA delivery system.

By specifying the bolus dose, lockout interval and infusion rate, the physician has already restricted the patient in the total amount of drug available each hour. Example: Morphine bolus 1 mg, lockout interval 5 minutes, and an infusion rate of 0.5 mg per hour, restricts the patient to a maximum of 12.5 mg <u>per hour</u>. Specifying a maximum 4 hour limit allows the physician to set a lower limit that can be delivered to the patient during this period. If one contrasts this with typical i.m. orders of 7.5 - 12.5 mg of morphine every 3 - 4 hours p.r.n., it is easy to see why patients on i.m. narcotics may have inadequate pain control.

DISCONTINUING PCA:

After the first or second postoperative day, the decision to add oral analgesics is based on the following considerations:

1. The patient is off a continuous PCA infusion.
2. The patient is requesting 2 or less PCA boluses every 4 hours.
3. The patient is having no or minimal pain at rest, and
4. The patient is able to ambulate and tolerate oral fluids.

Oral analgesics such as acetaminophen with codeine (Tylenol # 3® 1 - 2 tablets p.o. every 3 - 4 hours prn) should be started and used as the first line analgesic, and the PCA used for any additional *breakthrough* pain requirements (Table 16.3). The PCA can be discontinued once the patient is requiring minimal PCA bolus doses and tolerating the oral analgesics. The average patient having major surgery requires PCA therapy for 2 - 3 days.

NEURAXIAL OPIOIDS:

Within the superficial layers of the substantia gelatinosa, located in the dorsal horn of the spinal cord, exists a dense population of opioid receptors. Their activation results in a decrease in the release of neurotransmitters, such as substance P, and a decrease in transmission of painful stimuli from peripheral pain fibers at the level of the spinal cord.

The direct administration of opioids into the CSF by a spinal needle is referred to as an *intrathecal opioid* injection. The anaesthetist usually adds the opioid to the spinal local anaesthetic administered prior to surgery. This results in a very high local concentration of opioid within the CSF. The opioid diffuses readily to the opioid receptors located within the substantia gelatinosa, to provide analgesia at the spinal level (figure 16.3). Hence, this technique selectively targets opioid receptors responsible for regulating pain transmission at the spinal level.

By using the intrathecal route, the blood brain barrier is bypassed and superior analgesia may be obtained by contrast to narcotics administered by the i.v. or i.m. narcotic routes. The intrathecal administration of 0.2 mg of morphine may provide excellent analgesia for up to 16 hours after a total hip (replacement) arthroplasty. A similar patient treated with i.v. PCA morphine may require a total of 60 mg of morphine for the same initial period, and still have inferior pain relief as compared to the patient who received spinal narcotics.

Subarachnoid and epidural opioids are active at both the spinal cord level and at higher CNS levels. A portion of the opioids administered in the intrathecal space at the lumbar level will migrate along with the CSF circulating back to the brainstem. As with parentally (i.v., or i.m.) administered narcotics, high concentrations of narcotics at the brainstem level can result in respiratory depression, sedation, nausea, vomiting and puritis. The concentration of the narcotic in the spinal fluid decreases with the distance it migrates. The greater the opioid's lipid solubility, the more is taken up at the spinal cord level. Consequently, less drug migrates to the brainstem. Morphine, for example, has a low lipid solubility, and hence, has a greater tendency to migrate towards the brainstem as compared with meperidine or fentanyl, which have higher lipid solubilities.

EPIDURAL OPIODS:

The placement of an epidural catheter, in the epidural space permits a continuous infusion, or repeat administrations, of analgesics and local anaesthetics for several days. Dilute concentrations of local anaesthetic may be combined with epidural opioids in an attempt to exploit the analgesic properties of both. Epidural morphine has been used clinically since 1980 and is now used commonly to control acute severe pain.

NON OPIOD ANALGESICS
FOR ACUTE PAIN:

The non steroidal anti-inflammatory drugs (NSAIDs) are the most frequently used analgesics for acute pain. They include drugs such as aspirin, ibuprofen, indomethacin, naproxen, and many more. One new drug in this class, recently introduced in North America, is ketorolac (Toradol®). Extensive experience with this drug in Europe and Australia for acute postoperative pain control, has documented what appears to be an acceptable patient safety profile. One of the major advantages of ketorolac is its ability to be given both orally, and parentally. This has an obvious advantage in postoperative patients who are unable to take oral medications, yet are experiencing narcotic side effects despite poor pain control.

When tissues are traumatized they release peripheral inflammatory mediators which sensitize and stimulate peripheral nociceptors. Non steroidal anti-inflammatory drugs inhibit the enzyme, cyclooxygenase, which is involved in the production of many of these inflammatory mediators, through the arachnidonic acid pathway (e.g., prostaglandin E_2). Non steroidal anti-inflammatory drugs may also inhibit prostaglandins that are involved at the spinal cord level in the creating a state known as central hyper-sensitization. In this case their anti-prostaglandin effect of NSAIDs mitigate this hypersensitivity state, thereby decreasing the perception of pain.

Table 16.3
Contraindications to NSAIDs**

- Allergy to ASA, or other NSAID. Relative contraindication when there is a history of asthma, nasal polyps, or angioedema.
- Renal insufficiency
- Congestive heart failure
- Peptic ulcer disease
- Active inflammatory bowel disease
- Pregnancy or lactation
- Bleeding disorders

When considering using NSAIDs for acute pain management, physicians should review their contraindications and potential side effects (see table 16.3). When indicated, NSAIDs may be prescribed for short term therapy (less than 4 - 5 days) as an adjunct to acute pain management. For examples of typical regimens using NSAIDs in managing acute and chronic pain states see Table 16.2.

In patients for whom NSAIDs are contraindicated, acetaminophen can be an effective alternative. Since it has only

NSAIDs

Indomethacin (Indocid®)	25 - 75 mg po q8hrs	Start with 25 mg q8hrs
	50 - 100 mg pr supp.	Max. 200 mg/day
Ibuprofen (Motrin®)	400 - 800 mg po q 6-8 hrs	
Ketorolac (Toradol®)	10 mg po q 4-6 hrs	Max. po 40 mg/day
	10 - 30 mg im q 4-6 hrs	Max. im 120 mg/day

Tricyclic Antidepressants (TCA's)

Amitriptyline (Elavil®)	25 - 100 mg qhs	Use with caution in
Imipramine (Tofranil®)	25 - 100 mg qhs	patients with glaucoma or
Doxepine HCL (Sinequan®)	25 - 100 mg qhs	urinary retention.

Combinations

Acetaminophen + Codeine††   1 - 2 tabs po q 4-6 hrs

††(Tylenol® # 1,2, and 3 contain 300 mg acetaminophen + 15 mg caffeine + 8, 15, and 30 mg of codeine per tablet. Tylenol # 4 contains acetaminophen 300 mg, no caffeine, and 60 mg of codeine per tablet.)

Narcotics Agonist - Antagonist

Pentazocine HCL (Talwin®)	50 - 100 mg po q 4hrs	Useful in patients
Pentazocine Lactate (Talwin®)	30 - 60 mg sc, im, iv q 4hrs	who cannot tolerate codeine.

Opioids

Morphine Sulfate	15 - 30 mg po q4hrs
Morphine	5 - 15 mg im, sc q4hrs
Meperidine HCL (Demerol®)	50 - 150 mg po, im, sc q 3 - 4 hrs
Codeine	30 - 60 mg po, im q3 - 4 hrs

Table 16.2 Opioid and adjuvant medications commonly used to treat acute or chronic pain. Non steroidal anti-inflammatory medications are useful in patients who experience side effects from opioid pain medications. The generic drugs listed are accompanied by examples of common trade names in brackets.

weak peripheral inhibiting effects on prostaglandin synthesis, it lacks the side effects and contraindications listed above for NSAIDs. Still, acetaminophen strongly inhibits central prostaglandin synthesis, which accounts for its analgesic and antipyretic effects. One common postoperative problem is headaches. While a multitude of etiologies may be responsible for postoperative headaches (including caffeine withdrawal), acetaminophen (325 - 650 mg p.o. or p.r. every 4 - 6 hours) is generally effective, while narcotics are often ineffective.

NON PHARMACOLOGICAL INTERVENTIONS FOR ACUTE PAIN MANAGEMENT:

Anaesthesiologists are physicians who specialize in applying their knowledge of pharmacology and physiology to anaesthesia and analgesia. This chapter has focussed on pharmacological mechanisms and interventions in the management of acute pain. Still, there exist other alternative means of pain control that can be employed successfully by themselves or in conjunction with the pharmacologic interventions outlined in this chapter.

Patients have unique responses to pain. This varies according to such factors as their emotional and cultural backgrounds, and previous pain experience. Clinicians should anticipate that patients who use opioid analgesics regularly, will have increased analgesic requirements in the perioperative period (narcotic tolerance).

Cognitive and behaviour interventions may influence a patient's pain experience. Useful techniques in managing pain include:

1. Education and instruction.
2. Relaxation exercises.
3. Imagery.
4. Laughter.
5. Music distraction.
6. Biofeedback.
7. Conversation with family, friends, medical personnel.

Physical agents useful in alleviating pain include:

1. Applying of heat or cold.
2. Massaging, exercising, and stretching.
3. Transcutaneous electrical nerve stimulation (TENS).
4. Acupuncture.

References:

1. Clinical Practice Guideline. Acute pain management: Operative or medical procedures and trauma. U.S. Department of health and human services. 1992.

2. White P.F. Use of PCA for management of acute pain. JAMA 259:(2) 243-7; 1988.

3. Austin K.L. et al. Multiple intramuscular injections: a major source of variability in analgesic response to meperidine. Pain 8: 47; 1980.

4. Laurito C.E. Recent developments in postoperative pain management. Curr Rev Clin Anesth 12(5) 37-44, 1991.

5. Lubenow T.R. et al. Management of acute postoperative pain. Clin Anesth UPDATES: Vol 3; No.4, 1992.

6. Cousins N. Anatomy of an illness as perceived by the patient. Bantam Books New York, N.Y. 1979.

Notes:

Notes:

CHAPTER 17

Chronic Pain

LINDA ROBINSON M.D., FRCPC

INTRODUCTION

Chronic pain induces a cascade of changes in the patient involving physical, emotional and psychosocial changes. These combine with neural imprinting in the CNS to greatly influence the perceived severity and the consequences of the ongoing pain.

Chronic pain is defined as "an unpleasant sensory and emotional experience associated with actual or potential tissue damage, or described in terms of such damage". International Association for the Study of Pain (IASP) 1979.

This chapter will focus on five common chronic pain syndromes.

I. Post Herpetic Neuralgia
II. Causalgia
III. Reflex Sympathetic Dystrophy
IV. Myofascial Pain Syndromes
V. Low Back Pain

While similar nociceptive pathways and stimuli described for acute pain in chapter 16 are also active in chronic pain, there are distinct differences between acute and chronic pain disorders. To examine these differences, let's look at the example of Corporal Robert Ross, whom you are asked to see on your medical rounds. Corporal Ross had his left leg amputated below the hip after a combat injury in Korea in 1952. On entering his room, you find a man distraught, diaphoretic and complaining of severe pain in his left lower leg and foot. Anxious to get some hands on experience, you proceed to examine the affected limb, only to find that you are more than 40 years late! Is Mr. Ross faking his pain? How can he be having pain in a leg that he doesn't have?

Corporal Ross has a condition known as "phantom limb pain". Phantom limb pain, post herpetic neuralgia, and trigeminal neuralgia are examples of central pain states. Unlike pain which we have all experienced secondary to mechanical, chemical or thermal injury, this form of pain arises within the central nervous system. In these states, trauma, infection, or other conditions have damaged nerve tissue, resulting in abnormal activity in the intermediate afferent neurons in the CNS (see figure 16.1 chapter 16). The patient perceives real pain is occurring even though there is no nociceptive stimulation.

Altered sleep habits, inability to concentrate, inability to function (work, recreation), as well as depression, and abnormal behavioural coping mechanisms are common sequelae of chronic pain states.

PAIN CLINICS:

To address the diagnostic and therapeutic complexity of chronic pain conditions, multidisciplinary clinics have been established involving individuals with a specific interest in these disorders. These units commonly staff anaesthesiologists, psychologists, nurses and occupational or physical therapists. In addition, they have direct access to medical and surgical specialists, and various diagnostic services.

I: POST HERPETIC NEURALGIA

Acute Herpes Zoster (shingles) is a mononeuropathy caused by the reactivation of the Varicella-Zoster virus (VZV). Varicella is commonly known as chicken pox. This extremely contagious infection is usually seen as a benign illness in childhood. The VZV may lie dormant in the dorsal root ganglion for decades. When reactivated it presents as pain followed by a vesicular rash in the dermatomal distribution of the dorsal root ganglia involved. The disease presents as dermatomal pain which precedes the rash by 2 - 3 days. The rash is a maculopapular rash which evolves into vesicular lesions. The viral reactivation causes an acute hemorrhagic inflammation with demyelination and axonal degeneration. The damage to the nerve and root is permanent and of variable severity.

These patients suffer with constant severe burning pain. The area is exquisitely painful and they cannot bear even allowing their own clothes to touch them. This is frequently described as the worst pain they have ever experienced in their lives and the unremitting nature of the pain is very demoralizing and can lead to suicide in extreme cases. Normally the total duration of the disease is between 7 to 10 days, with the skin returning to normal within 2 to 4 weeks.

The most debilitating complication of herpes zoster is the development of post herpetic neuralgia. While this complication is extremely uncommon in young individuals, it occurs in 50% of patients over the age of 50 with zoster. Typically the patient experiences gradual improvement over several weeks. However some patients may be left with a chronic life long neuralgic pain. After about 6 - 8 weeks, the pain of herpes zoster is called Post Herpetic Neuralgia. The chance of a patient developing post herpetic neuralgia increases steadily with age.

TREATMENT

Various treatments may be considered for herpes zoster, although none is entirely satisfactory. The acute Herpes Zoster can be treated with an antiviral agent such as Acyclovir (Zovirax®), but to be of any help this agent must be initiated immediately upon making the diagnosis. Unfortunately, Acyclovir treatment is very expensive; a typical course can run over $1000. Even though it may shorten the acute phase of H.Z. and result in lesions healing earlier, there is no evidence that it prevents post herpetic neuralgia.

Optimal treatment depends upon accurate diagnosis. Frequently, however, patients present with pain before the rash develops, resulting in an incorrect diagnosis. Common diagnosis at this stage include myocardial infarction, acute prolapsed disc, and kidney stones. Acute pain should be treated as soon as possible. Physicians often use narcotics, but these are less effective for treating neuralgic pain than other pain disorders. Narcotics may, however, 'take the edge' off the pain and make it more tolerable. Better still, nerve blocks can provide temporary or permanent relief without the risk of the narcotic dependency. Infiltrating the area with a dilute local anesthetic and steroid has also been used successfully, and requires little technical skill on the part of the physician.

In the chronic phase some patients still require acetaminophen with codeine (Tylenol No. 3®) or a stronger narcotic. Still, other drugs (tricyclic antidepressants (TCAs) and anticonvulsants, discussed below) are usually more effective. As with the other chronic pain syndromes, the sooner treatment is initiated, the more effective it is.

A tricyclic antidepressant is frequently used as a first line drug in treating post herpetic neuralgia. Nevertheless care must be taken to monitor for side effects. These patients are frequently elderly, and prone to becoming confused, dizzy, or developing urinary retention as a result of the anticholinergic activity of TCA's.

Anticonvulsants such as phenytoin (dilantin®), and carbamazepine (tegretol®) have also been used with some success. Capsaicin (zostrix®) cream is a relatively new treatment designed specifically for this problem. It contains capsaicin which depletes the neurotransmitter substance P in the peripheral nerve endings and results in a decrease in nociceptive information.

Some patients respond well to transcutaneous electrical nerve stimulation (TENS), which is particularly useful in elderly patients because it has few side effects. By stimulating the large diameter nerve fibres, smaller fibres carrying painful stimuli at the level of the dorsal horn are inhibited, according to the Gate theory of pain.

Mexilitene HCL, an oral 1b anti arrhythmic with properties similar to lidocaine, has also be used to alleviate this form of neuralgic pain. Despite utilizing all these modalities, post herpetic neuralgia sometimes remains resistant to medical treatment.

II. CAUSALGIA

Causalgia is a painful disorder associated with injury of the peripheral nerves. In 1864, Wier Mitchell presented a treatise entitled, "Gunshot wounds and other injuries of nerves". In this paper he describes an injured unionist soldier as follows:

In our early experience of nerve wounds, we met with a small number of men who were suffering from a pain which they described as 'burning' or as 'mustard red-hot' or as a 'red hot file rasping the skin'....it never attacks the trunk, rarely the arm or thigh....its favoured site is the foot or hand....the part itself becomes exquisitely hyperaesthetic, so that a touch or a tap of the finger increases the pain. Exposure to the air is avoided by the patient with a care which seems absurd, and most of the bad cases keep the hand constantly wet, finding relief from the wet....As the pain increases the temper changes and grows irritable, and the face becomes anxious, and has a look of weariness and suffering. The sleep is restless....and exasperates the hyperaesthetic state so that the rattling of a newspaper, a breath of fresh air, the step across the ward, or the shock of the feet in walking, gives rise to increase of pain.

Mitchell, provides a classical description of the deep red, glossy, and mottled trophic skin changes that characterize this pain syndrome. He used the term "causalgia" to describe these changes. World wars I and II left many soldiers with these traumatic causalgic pain disorders. Since then, centres studying these peripheral nerve injuries note that victims of high velocity missile injuries involving the brachial plexus or sciatic nerve plexus, are at risk of developing this chronic pain disorder.

The pain is aggravated by a variety of physical and emotional factors frequently leading to profound emotional, physical and behavioural disturbances. In the late stages of the disorder, vasomotor (circulatory) and sudomotor (sweat gland) changes accompany trophic skin changes.

If the sympathetic nerves to the affected limb can be interrupted soon after the injury, prompt and complete relief of the pain can be obtained. Occasionally, spontaneous remission occurs, but without treatment most patients progress to develop irreversible trophic changes in the affected limb. The lower incidence of these changes among Vietnam Veterans (1.5%) compared to WW II Veterans (5 - 10%) is probably due to the more rapid treatment of injuries with early debridement in Vietnam.

Causalgia usually involves the median, sciatic or brachial plexus nerves, because they carry the bulk of sensory and sympathetic fibres. Nevertheless, identical syndromes have developed in patients suffering trigeminal, occipital, and intercostal nerve injuries.

CHARACTERISTICS OF CAUSALGIC PAIN:

Most patients develop causalgic pain within a week of the injury. They experience a burning superficial pain in the periphery of the extremity, most intense in the fingers and palm, or toes and sole. The pain is so intense and persistent, it overwhelms patients, prohibiting rest, sleep, and resulting in profound psychological disturbances.

One study, using the McGill Pain Questionnaire, found a rating scale of 42 (out of 50) in causalgia, as compared to 25 for phantom limb pain, 26 for back pain and cancer pain, and 23 for Post Herpetic Neuralgia (see figure 17.1). Two thirds of patients also describe a deep, intermittent stabbing, tearing, or crushing pain.

Initially, the pain is located in the general territory of the nerve, but as the syndrome progresses it spreads to involve areas well beyond the affected nerve's distribution.

Passive movement of the part, light touch, loud noises, or emotional outbursts aggravate the pain. Even clothes or bed sheets are unbearable, and patients go to any length to avoid moving the part.

SENSORY AND MOTOR DISTURBANCES

Allodynia (see glossary of terms at the end of the chapter) to touch and temperature develop as does hyperpathia. Vasodilation occurs early followed by vasoconstriction.

Trophic changes develop and the affected part becomes red and glossy with denuded skin, tapering digits, and coarse rigid nails. The small interphalangeal joints stiffen and become fixed, muscles atrophy and eventually develop contractions. The trophic changes can be avoided if treatment is instituted within 1-2 months of the injury.

Psychologically, the individual may manifest bizarre behaviourial changes, with limb guarding, and seclusion. These changes are reversible if the pain is treated adequately.

Treatment options clinicians utilize for this disorder include:

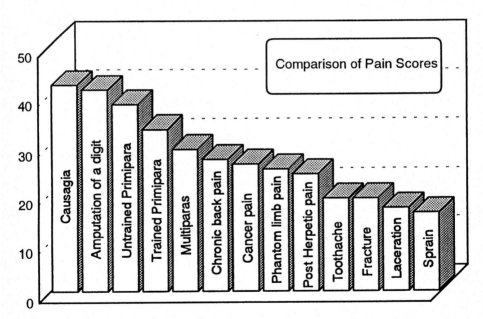

Figure 17.1: Comparison of pain scores of common pain conditions using the McGill Pain Questionairre. Modified with permission from Melzack R. Psychological aspects of pain: implications for neural blockade. In Neural blockade. Cousins MJ, Bridenbaugh PO. (eds) 2nd edit. J.B. Lippincott Co. 1988.

1. Sympathetic blockade with local anaesthetics or other agents (see 1a and 1b below). This is frequently useful as a diagnostic tool, however, patients who fail to respond may have a condition called "Sympathetic Independent Pain".

1a. Local anesthetic blocks of either the stellate ganglion (for the arm), or the lumbar sympathetic plexus (for the leg).

1b. A "Bier Block" (see chapter 16, figure 16.4) with iv guanethidine or reserpine has also been used to produce a localized sympathectomy.

These blocks must be repeated to achieve lasting effect. Guanethidine displaces norepinephrine from stores in the sympathetic nerve endings and also prevents the reuptake of norepinephrine. This results in the loss of sympathetic adrenergic nerve function for days or weeks.

2. Oral alpha 1 adrenergic blockers, such as phenoxybenzamine, can be used as a means of decreasing the excessive sympathetic barrage present in causalgic pain disorders. Side effects are nausea and postural hypotension.

3. Chemical sympathectomy may be created by the administration of local anaesthetics or other agents (see 1a, 1b). If a chemical sympathectomy is effective in providing temporary relief, the clinician may recommend a surgical sympathectomy for these patients, in the hope of effecting a permanent cure. Unfortunately, surgical sympathectomy is not always successful, and the pain may recur.

4. Others modalities that have proved useful in treating this condition include TENS, dorsal column stimulation, physical therapy, and psychotherapy.

III: REFLEX SYMPATHETIC DYSTROPHY *

Reflex sympathetic dystrophy (RSD) is a term for a variety of conditions including: minor causalgia, post traumatic pain syndrome, Sudeck's atrophy, and shoulder hand syndrome.

The precipitating factors include accidental or surgical trauma, and a variety of disease states. Pain, vasomotor changes, autonomic disturbances, delayed recovery of function and trophic changes characterize RSD. Early treatment with sympathetic interruption results in pain relief and reverses the pathophysiological abnormalities.

Compared to causalgia, a reflex sympathetic dystrophy is a more common outcome of orthopaedic injuries and industrial accidents. Hence, it must be promptly recognized and treated.

The most common cause of RSD is trauma (e.g., sprains, dislocations, fractures, crush injuries, and lacerations). There is no correlation between the severity of original injury and the development of RSD. Even a Colles fracture resulting in a minor peripheral nerve injury can result in RSD.

Reflex sympathetic dystrophy is one complication of common surgical procedures (e.g., amputations, excision of ganglia, tight casts, carpal tunnel release). It may also be due to an underlying medical condition such as a myocardial infarction (shoulder-hand syndrome), or diabetes (diabetic neuropathy). Direct nerve compression from a herniated disc, tumours of spine, or metastases compressing the branchial plexus may also result in RSD.

In contrast with causalgia, where pain develops rapidly, the pain of RSD develops over weeks or months after the injury.

The criteria for a diagnosis of RSD are:

1.   There is a history of recent or remote accidental or iatrogenic trauma or disease.

2.   The patient complains of a persistent pain that is burning, aching or throbbing.

3.   One or more of:
    a.   vasomotor/sudomotor changes
    b.   trophic changes, edema, hypersensitivity to cold
    c.   muscle weakness, or atrophy

4.   Relief of symptoms is obtained after regional sympathetic blockade.

TREATMENT OF RSD *:

Original injuries should receive proper and rapid treatment (including removal of foreign bodies, immobilization, repair of muscles and tendons, and pain relief) in the hope of preventing the subsequent development of RSD.

Treatment modalities include the early use of sympathetic blocks, physiotherapy, psychotherapy, medical therapy (eg. phenoxybenzamine, prednisone), and, when these fail, a surgical sympathectomy.

IV: MYOFASCIAL PAIN SYNDROME *

This chronic pain syndrome comprises a large group of muscle disorders characterized by the presence of hypersensitive points (called trigger points) producing pain, muscle spasm, tenderness, stiffness, and weakness.

Various terms such as fibrositis, fibromyositis, and muscular rheumatism have been used to describe the myofascial pain syndrome. The condition is most commonly misdiagnosed as bursitis, arthritis, visceral disease, or a herniated disc.

Trauma to the myofascial structures and an acute overload on the affected muscles is the most common cause of this syndrome. Acute muscle strain damages the sarcoplasmic reticulum releasing excessive amounts of calcium. This initiates a complex cascade of events beginning with local vasoconstriction, sustained muscular contraction, decreased blood flow, increased metabolism, and culminating in the release of nerve sensitizing substances. In the affected areas, taut muscle bands may be palpable and are referred to as trigger points. Pain from myofascial trigger points (TP's) is described as steady, deep, and aching. The pain may be exacerbated by stretch, cold, stress, fatigue, viral illnesses or direct pressure.

An acute episode of myofascial pain often follows overuse of unconditioned muscles (e.g., the weekend athlete), poor posture during prolonged activities such as computer work, or automobile accidents (whiplash).

Patients present with persistent pain, tight or aching muscles, limited range of

Table 17.1 Comparison of Causalgia and Reflex Sympathetic Dystrophy.

	Causalgia	RSD
Onset	Within 1 week	Over weeks to months
Frequency	Rare	More common
Etiology	Typically involves high velocity injuries of the brachial or sciatic nerve plexus (e.g., gun shot wounds).	Accidental injuries, surgical trauma, orthopaedic injuries (e.g., sprain, fracture, tight cast, dislocation).
Pain Characteristics	Similar pain characteristics, typically described as a constant burning, throbbing, or aching pain. Disturbed sleep, and profound psychological-behavioural changes are more common with causalgia. The affected limb is guarded, and becomes cool, pale or cyanotic, accompanied by decreased hair growth, muscle atrophy, tendon contracture, and joint ankylosis. Causalgia is generally recognized as the most intense form of chronic pain, and has a McGill Pain Score average of 42/50 (see figure 17.1).	
Prevention	Early treatment of the injury with debridement, repair and immobilization of associated fractures.	

Treatment	Sympathetic blocks:
	    Stellate ganglion block (arm),
	    Lumbar sympathetic block (leg)
	    Guanethidine intravenous Bier block (see figure 15.4)
	Alpha-1 adrenergic blockers (e.g., phenoxybenzamine)
	Other:
	    Physical therapy, psychotherapy, TENS,
	    dorsal column stimulation, surgical sympathectomy.	

motion and generalized fatigue. They may experience continuous or intermittent muscular pains, aches or a burning sensation in the overloaded muscles. Applying direct pressure on these trigger points exacerbates the pain. Predictable patterns of pain associated with specific TP's do not follow a dermatomal distribution.

For effective treatment, the pain and spasm cycle must be interrupted. The TP can be injected with local anaesthetic, or the overlying skin sprayed with a vaporized coolant. These treatments should be followed by stretching of the affected muscle groups.

Patients are frequently in poor physical condition and should slowly but methodically undertake a program of progressive daily physical fitness. This should include aerobic exercises, such as walking, exercise biking, swimming, low impact aerobics and aqua fitness. Physician's may motivate patients by reminding them that this is the most important aspect of their treatment.

These patients frequently have very poor sleep patterns. Tricyclic antidepressants in low doses will improve sleep and decrease the level of muscular pain (possibly by increasing serotonin levels). Cyclobenzaprine HCL (Flexeril®) is also commonly used as a 'skeletal muscle relaxant'. As this tends to be a chronic condition, narcotics should be avoided due to the risk of opioid dependence. Plain acetaminophen can be used instead.

V: LOW BACK PAIN *

Low back pain is one of the most common problems our society faces. Sixty to eighty percent of all adults will suffer with this at least once during their lifetime. The pain is usually self limited. Of those who see their doctor, more than 90% will improve and are back to work within 2 months. However, the remaining 5-10% pose a challenging problem.

Risk Factors for low back pain include:
Increasing age
Heavy labour
Lower education and income
Smoking
Obesity
Whole body vibration (truck driver)
Previous back pain

A host of clinical entities have been described to explain the various types of low back pain, such as muscle strain, degenerative disc disease, facet syndrome, and myofascial pain syndrome. However, the signs, symptoms and radiological findings of these conditions overlap, making an accurate diagnosis difficult. For example, a patient who, on clinical examination, appears to have facet joint pain and degenerative disc disease, may nevertheless have similar radiological changes to other patients who are entirely asymptomatic.

Low back pain is usually not an emergency. Occasionally, conditions** do present as low back pain and may have dire consequences for a patient should the clinician fail to make the correct diagnosis.

Table 17.2:	Causes of Low Back Pain

(Ninety percent of all cases of back pain are due to "medical causes")

Medical Conditions

Musculoskeletal:
- Muscle 'strain'
- Ligament 'sprain'
- Apophyseal joint: 'facet syndrome'
- Discs: 'degenerative disc disease'
- Bone: fractures, spondylolisthesis

Neoplastic:
- Benign: osteoid osteoma
- Malignant
  Primary: Multiple myeloma
  Secondary: Metastasis

Infectious:
- Acute: pyogenic discitis, osteomyelitis
- Chronic tuberculosis

Inflammatory:
- Ankylosing spondylitis
- Psoriatic spondylitis
- Reactive arthritis
- Inflammatory bowel disease

Metabolic:
- Osteoporosis $\pm$ fractures
- Osteomalacia
- Paget's disease of the bone

Visceral:
- Pelvic organs
  (endometriosis, prostatitis)
- Renal disease (pyelonephritis)
- Gastrointestinal disorder
  (pancreatitis, peptic ulcer)
- Aortic aneurysm

Surgical Emergencies (see text)
- Cauda Equina Syndrome (disc herniation, tumor mass, abscess)
- Aortic aneurysm (leaking, dissecting, ruptured)

Sciatica with Neurologic Signs
- Ruptured intervertebral disc
- Spinal stenosis

For example, the cauda equina syndrome presents as a constellation of symptoms and signs such as a neurologic deficit in the lower extremities (paralysis and loss of sensation), loss of bowel or bladder continence, weakness, depressed reflexes, and loss of sensation over the buttocks called "saddle anaesthesia". This is a surgical emergency and rapid decompression of the spinal cord is needed to avoid permanent nerve damage. Causes of cauda equina syndrome include central disc herniation, and epidural tumours or abscesses.

An aortic aneurysm may present as back pain and may require immediate surgical attention. Sciatica is usually caused by a herniated disc or by a narrow spinal canal with compression of the nerve roots (spinal stenosis). The patient experiences pain that radiates below the knee. A herniated disc tends to be aggravated by prolonged sitting, or anything that increases intrathecal pressure (eg. sneezing, or coughing). Paresthesia and weakness may be experienced in the involved nerve root distribution.

Spinal stenosis is more common in patients over 60 years of age. Characteristically, these patients complain of pain in the buttocks, thighs and legs, which develops on standing and walking, and is relieved by 15-20 minutes of rest. Patients find that walking with the trunk flexed is more comfortable.

Other medical causes presenting as sciatica include tumours, infection, and arthritis.

Conservative treatment of sciatica with rest, analgesics, nonsteroidal anti inflammatory medications, muscle relaxants, or epidural steroids is usually sufficient, (provided other more serious conditions have been excluded - see Table 17.2). Surgery is indicated if persistent disabling pain occurs or the neurologic deficit increases despite conservative measures.

The treatment of 'medical back pain' should be specific to the medical condition. A tumour with metastasis to the spine may require surgical intervention, chemotherapy or radiotherapy.

Osteo-myelitis may require antibiotics and drainage. Arthritis requires specific treatment for the underlying disease.

Mechanical low back pain is managed with a several days of rest, oral analgesics, NSAID's, and then mobilization. Chronic low back pain is frequently difficult to treat and requires a gradual program of aerobic conditioning, physiotherapy, tricyclic antidepressants, psychotherapy and education about proper back care.

GLOSSARY OF TERMS:

Allodynia: Pain due to a stimulus that does not normally provide pain.

Analgesia: Absence of pain in response to stimulation that would normally be painful.

Causalgia: A syndrome of sustained burning pain, allodynia, and hyperpathia after a traumatic nerve lesion, often combined with vasomotor and sudomotor dysfunction and later trophic changes.

Dysesthesia: An unpleasant abnormal sensation, whether spontaneous or evoked.

Hyperalgesia: An increased response to a stimulus that is normally painful.

Hyperesthesia: Increased sensitivity to stimulation, excluding the special senses.

Hyperpathia: A painful syndrome, characterized by increased reaction to a stimulus, especially a repetitive stimulus, as well as an increased threshold.

Hypoalgesia: Diminished pain response to normally painful stimulus.

Hypoesthesia: Decreased sensitivity to stimulation, excluding the special senses.

Neuralgia: Pain in the distribution of a nerve or nerves.

Neuritis: Inflammation of a nerve or nerves.

Neuropathy: A disturbance of function or pathological change in a nerve; in one nerve, mononeuropathy; in several nerves, mononeuropathy multiplex; if diffuse and bilateral, polyneuropathy.

Nociceptor: A receptor preferentially sensitive to a noxious stimulus or to a stimulus that would become noxious if prolonged.

Pain tolerance level: The greatest level of pain that a subject is prepared to tolerate.

Pain threshold: The least experience of pain that a subject can recognize.

Paresthesia: An abnormal sensation, whether spontaneous or evoked.

CHAPTER 18

Obstetrical Anaesthesia

ROBERT ELLIOT MD FRCPC

This chapter will focus on the following four topics:

1. The physiological changes of pregnancy and their clinical significance.
2. The importance of the supine hypotensive syndrome and aortocaval compression.
3. Available options for providing pain relief during labour and delivery, including epidural analgesia.
4. The risks of general anaesthesia in the parturient.

I: Physiological Changes*.

For anaesthetic interventions in the parturient, one must consider both the physiological changes that occur during pregnancy, as well as the effects of anaesthetic drugs on the mother and infant. Complications during labour and delivery may threaten the life of both the parturient and her infant. The anaesthetist must be able to respond quickly, working closely with the obstetric, neonatal, and nursing teams.

Profound physiological changes occur during pregnancy. Changes in the nervous, cardiorespiratory, and gastrointestinal systems, and their implications with respect to the anaesthetic management, are reviewed in tables 18.1 - 18.3.

II: Supine Hypotensive Syndrome**:

The gravid uterus may compress the inferior vena cava (IVC), and/or the aorta when the parturient lies in the supine position. This occurs in approximately 15% of patients as early as the 20th week, and increases in frequency in the third trimester.

When IVC compression results from uterine compression, there is a decrease in venous return to the heart. The parturient may experience signs and symptoms of shock including hypotension, pallor, sweating, nausea, vomiting and changes in mentation. Venous pressure in the lower extremities and in the uterus increases. Blood flow to the uterus occurs because of a difference between the uterine artery and venous pressures. Hence an increase in uterine venous pressure will decrease the uterine blood flow to the placenta and fetus.

Compression of the aorta by itself, is not associated with maternal hypotension, but, may result in arterial hypotension in the uterus. This decrease in uterine blood flow may result in fetal distress or asphyxia.

Table 18.1	The physiological changes of pregnancy.		
Nervous System			
Variable	**Change**	**Cause**	**Importance**
General Anaesthesia	MAC Requirements decrease by 25 - 40%	CNS effect of progesterone and (or) beta-endorphin	General anaesthetic drug requirements are decreased.
Regional Anaesthesia	Local Anaesthetic (LA) dose requirements decrease by about 40%	Decrease in size of epidural space due to engorged epidural veins, and (or) hormonal changes.	Increased epidural spread of LA may occur, esp. if aorto-caval compression is not prevented.
Cardiovascular System			
Blood Volume (BV)	Total BV ↑ by 35% Plasma BV ↑ by 45% RBC's BV ↑ by 20%	Hormonal effect	An ↑ of approx. 1000 ml compensates for the 400 - 600 ml of blood loss with delivery.
Cardiac Output (CO)	↑ by 40% at 10 weeks gestation labour ↑ CO 45% above pre-labour values. After delivery CO ↑ 60% above pre-labour values.	Increases in CO are in response to increased meta-bolic demands. (Stroke volume increases more than heart rate).	Patients with pre-existing heart disease may decompensate. (eg. Pulm. edema may occur during labour or after deliv-ery in the patient with significant mitral stenosis).
Peripheral Circulation	BP normal or ↓ SVR ↓ by 15%. Venous return from legs decreases.	SVR decreases to compensate for ↑ in CO, leaving BP normal or ↓.	Supine Hypotensive Syndrome. (see text)
Regional Blood Flow	Uterus increases blood flow by 500 ml / min.	Blood flow in the placenta is dependent on blood pressure.	Placental blood flow cannot ↑ but can ↓ with maternal ↓ BP due to blood loss, aortocaval compression, or catecholamines.

Table 18.2   The physiological changes of pregnancy (continued).

Respiratory System

Variable	Change	Cause	Importance
Upper Airway	Mucosal edema makes the parturient prone to bleeding.	Capillary engorgement.	Trauma may occur with suctioning, and placing nasal or oral airways. Choose a smaller ETT.
Ventilation	Minute Ventilation increases by 50%. Tidal volume ↑ 40%. Respiratory rate ↑ 10%.	Increases in O_2 consumption begins in the first trimester. Labour may increase O_2 consumption more than 100%.	Normal resting maternal $PaCO_2$ drops to approx. 30 mm Hg in the first trimester. Pain from labour and delivery result in further hyperventilation.
Lung Volumes	FRC ↓ 20%. No change in V.C.	By fifth month the rising uterus begins to force the diaphragm up.	Uptake of inhaled anaesthetics occurs faster due to increased minute ventilation with a smaller FRC.
Arterial Oxygenation PaO_2	Increased by 10 mm Hg.	Due to hyperventilation.	Decreased FRC with increased O_2 consumption result in very rapid decreases in PaO_2 during apnea (eg. induction of general anaesthesia). Pulse oximetry is important.

The term parturient should never be placed in the supine position. Abnormal fetal heart rate patterns indicating insufficient uterine blood flow are frequently observed when patients are placed in the supine position (see figure 18.1). Positioning the parturient on her side, or using a 10 - 15 cm right hip wedge is usually sufficient to move the weight of the uterus off the IVC and aorta. Lumbar regional anaesthetics block the sympathetic nerves and decrease vascular tone in the lower body. This may exaggerate the hypotensive effects of aortocaval compression.

Table 18.3	The physiological changes of pregnancy (continued).		
Gastrointestinal System			
Variable	Change	Cause	Importance
Gastric Fluid Volume	Increased	Enlarged uterus displaces pylorus. Gastric emptying delayed.	**N.B.** All parturients are considered to have a "**full stomach**". Pain, anxiety and drugs (esp. narcotics) all retard gastric emptying. Metoclopramide may be useful in reducing volume. (see chapter 9: The rapid sequence induction)
Gastric Fluid Acidity	Increased	Gastrin secreted by placenta. Stimulates H+ secretion.	Use of H2-receptor antagonists (ranitidine) and (or) a non-particulate antacid (Na citrate) are recommended to increase gastric pH.
Gastro-esophageal junction.	Decreased competence.	Enlarging uterus distorts the angle of the junction.	Pulm. aspiration of gastric contents is the major risk of Gen. Anaesthesia. Placement of an ETT is mandatory in every parturient rendered unconscious by anaesthesia. (see chapter 24: Unusual Anaesthetic Complications: Aspiration Syndrome).

III: Analgesia options for Labour and Delivery.**

How painful is labour?

The pain of labour is generally described as being more intense than any other previous pain experience (see chapter 17 figure 17.1: Comparison of common pain conditions). In women delivering for the first time, the pain of labour is described as more intense than the pain of their subsequent labours. During labour nociceptive impulses resulting from labour and delivery are transmitted from **visceral** nerve fibres entering the spinal cord at **T10 to L1**. During delivery somatic nociceptive impulses enter the spinal cord at **S2 to S4**, see figure 18.2. Table 18.4 lists some of the factors which influence the degree and intensity of the pain experience during labour.

Psychoprophylaxis: The Lamaze method postulates that the parturient's pain which arises from uterine contractions and perineal distension can be replaced with conditioned "positive" reflexes. This method uses a partner or friend who functions as a coach helping the parturient concentrate on breathing techniques and on releasing muscle tension. Emphasis is placed on education about labour and delivery, to give the parturient a sense of "control" over the birth process. Some proponents of the Lamaze method advocate not using any chemical anaesthesia for fear of placental transfer to the fetus. Psychoprophylaxis reduces the need for "chemical anaesthesia", however studies have shown that two-thirds of Lamaze mothers will require some kind of analgesic aid. Furthermore, it is unfair to suggest that, if the method is followed correctly, labour will be painless. This can only lower self-esteem when "failure" occurs.

In fact, excessive pain may result in more harm to the fetus than the judicious use of pharmacologic analgesia. Psychologic stress during labour may cause hypoxia and acidosis in the fetus.

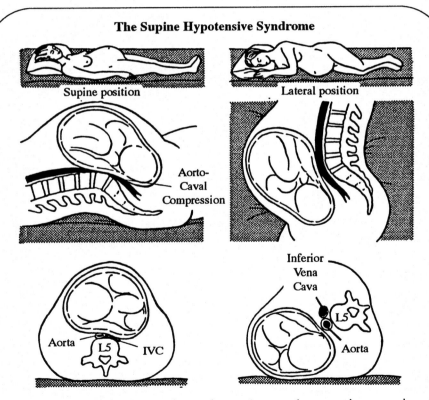

The Supine Hypotensive Syndrome

Supine position

Lateral position

Aorto-Caval Compression

Inferior Vena Cava

L5

Aorta

L5

IVC

Aorta

Figure 18.1: The supine hypotensive syndrome. Aortocaval compression occurs in the supine position and is relieved by positioning the parturient in the lateral position. (Adapted with permission from Bonica JJ: Obstetric Analgesia and Anesthesia. World Federation of Societies of Anaesthesiologists, Amsterdam, 1980.)

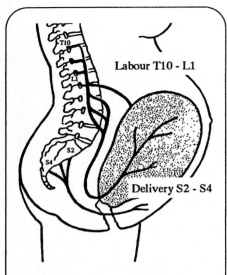

Labour T10 - L1

Delivery S2 - S4

Figure 18.2: Nociceptive pathways in labour and delivery.

Table 18.4: Factors influencing the pain of labour and delivery*.

- Parturient's psychological state
- Mental preparation
- Family support
- Medical support
- Cultural background
- Primipara vs. multipara
- Size and presentation of the fetus
- Size and anatomy of the pelvis
- Use of medications to augment labour (eg. oxytocin)
- Duration of labour

This is believed to result from decreased uterine blood flow secondary to elevated levels of blood catecholamines and (or) decreased carbon dioxide tensions caused by hyperventilation. With adequate pain relief, epidural anaesthesia can minimize the stress of labour, and facilitate patient participation during labour and delivery. It is important to recognize differences in pain tolerance and analgesic requirements in order to promote maternal self-esteem and bonding with the newborn.

Table 18.5 lists some of the options currently available for pain management during labour. Table 18.6 lists some of the pharmacokinetic properties of two opioids used in managing pain during labour and delivery.

Meperidine is transferred very quickly across the placenta. However, peak levels in the fetus are not reached until 2 to 3 hours after administration. Therefore, infants born 2 - 3 hours after maternal meperidine administration are at risk of opioid-induced depression. Elimination of meperidine from the neonate takes 3 - 6 days. Normeperidine, an active metabolite, takes even longer and may be responsible for subtle behavioral changes in the newborn infant.

Fentanyl is transferred to the fetus extremely rapidly and redistributes back to the mother, much like thiopental. With doses of 1 mcg/kg, fentanyl does not produce adverse effects on the neonate, and is eliminated from the fetus much quicker than meperidine.

Table 18.5:	Options available for pain management during labour and delivery**.

- Nothing
- Psychological support (coaches, husband, family members)
- Behavioral modification (Lamaze technique)
- Hypnotherapy (relaxation exercises practised in months prior to L&D).
- Education (normal expectations for labour and delivery; prenatal classes).
- Massage, walking.
- Sedatives.
- Opioid analgesics (e.g., meperidine p.o., i.m., i.v., fentanyl i.v.).
- Opioid - antiemetic combinations
  (e.g., meperidine 50 - 100 mg with dimenhydrinate [Gravol] 50 mg i.m.).
- Epidural analgesia (local anaesthesia alone, or with epidural opioids
  e.g., bupivacaine 0.125% with fentanyl 2 mcg/ml).
- Spinal anaesthesia (see text for discussion).
- General anaesthesia (see text for discussion).

Table 18.7 reviews some of the potential maternal and neonatal advantages of epidural analgesia. The recommended doses, complications and contraindications to epidural analgesia and anaesthesia were presented in chapter 15: Local and regional anaesthesia.

Lidocaine and bupivacaine are the most common local anaesthetic agents used for managing epidural analgesia - anaesthesia. Low concentrations of bupivacaine (e.g. 0.125%) can provide a differential nerve block (see chapter 15). This results in only a minor motor nerve block. As a consequence, the patient maintains her motor strength, permitting her to move during labour. During the second stage of labour, the differential nerve block facilitates her efforts to push, by minimizing the motor block while maintaining an adequate sensory block.

Epinephrine is frequently added to the LA (e.g. 1:200,000 epinephrine or 5 mcg/ml). This can increase the duration of nerve blockade by 50%, decrease the

Opioid Agonist	Dose	Peak Effect	Duration
Meperidine (Demerol®)	PO 50 - 150 mg. IM 50 -150 mg. IV 25 mg.	1 - 1½ hours 40 - 50 mins. 5 - 10 mins.	2 - 4 hours
Fentanyl (Sublimaze®)	IM 50 - 100 mcg. IV 25 - 50 mcg.	IM 7 - 8 mins. IV 3 - 5 mins.	0.5 - 1 hour

Table 18.6: Common opioid analgesics for labour and delivery.

Epidural Analgesia - Anaesthesia.	
Maternal Advantages.	**Neonatal advantages.**
1. **Excellent pain relief,** frequently achieved compared to opioids alone. 2. **Normal progress of labour** once established is not impeded. 3. **General anaesthesia avoided,** should a Caesarean section, or forceps manipulation be required (epidural level is increased for C-section). 4. **Improved maternal participation** in delivery and during bonding with the newborn.	1. **Less drug transfer** to the infant, due to a decrease in maternal sedatives and opioid requirements. 2. **Improved uterine blood flow** and fetal well being may result with the relief of the maternal stress response during labour and delivery. 3. **Reduced neonatal trauma** during delivery with improved conditions when the use of forceps is required. 4. **No neonatal depression,** when properly managed.

Table 18.7: Epidural anaesthesia in labour and delivery.

systemic absorption by 30%, and decrease the overall amount of drug required. Epinephrine is believed to cause vasoconstriction of the epidural blood vessels, decreasing the drug's systemic uptake. Potential side effects of adding epinephrine include a significant increase in motor block, accentuation of hypertension in preeclamptic patients, and diminished uterine activity due to the beta-effects of epinephrine.

Spinal anaesthesia is generally not used for labour and delivery because of the intense motor block it creates, making pushing during stage II ineffective. As spinal anaesthesia is usually provided by one injection, it lacks the flexibility in duration that can be achieved by using a continuous epidural catheter.

While general anaesthesia for labour and delivery was used in the pioneer days of anaesthesia, our understanding of the risks of general anaesthesia to both the mother and neonate has made this mode of analgesia obsolete.

IV: General Anaesthesia.
When regional anaesthesia is contraindicated, or there is insufficient time to establish regional anaesthesia (e.g. severe sustained fetal bradycardia), general anaesthesia for operative delivery may be required. The anaesthetist faced with providing general anaesthesia for Caesarean section must consider the physiological changes of pregnancy, and be ready to provide care for the compromised neonate. Immediate concerns include*:

1. All parturients must be considered to have a *"full stomach"* and gastric precautions including a *rapid sequence induction* with cricoid pressure are indicated for general anaesthesia.
2. Upper airway edema occurs with pregnancy and all parturients should be considered to have a potentially *difficult airway* to intubate.
3. General anaesthesia introduces the risks of a failed intubation, and the risk of *hypoxemia*, and/or pulmonary *aspiration* of gastric acid.
4. With general anaesthesia we must consider the potential of having maternal drugs transferred to the neonate. This may contribute to *neonatal depression* and the need for neonatal resuscitation.

The 'rapid sequence induction' was presented in chapter 9. In the pregnant patient with a potentially difficult airway, a thorough evaluation of the airway is especially important (see chapter 6). All parturients have a tendency to rapid desaturation with induction of general anaesthesia. Hence 'pre-oxygenation' with 100% oxygen prior to induction of general anaesthesia is critically important for all parturients. Pre-oxygenation is provided with a properly sealed mask applied to the patient's face, with the patient breathing 100% oxygen. If the patient breathes 100% oxygen for ≥ 3 minutes, or takes four vital capacity breaths, more than 95% of the nitrogen in the patients FRC will be exchanged with oxygen. The normal resting FRC is approximately 2.5 litres, and contains 80% nitrogen. By replacing the nitrogen with oxygen, we provide a reserve of oxygen for the period of apnea that occurs during induction of anaesthesia.

A small dose of curare is often used in a 'rapid sequence induction' to prevent the intense muscle fasciculations that may occur following the administration of succinylcholine. In the pregnant patient, the muscle fasciculations are much less intense, probably due to the effect of progesterone. Many anaesthetists omit curare pretreatment in the obstetrical patient because it prolongs the onset time of succinylcholine paralysis and reduces the intensity of the neuromuscular block.

The difficult intubation:
On rare occasions, the anaesthetist may be unable to intubate the patient on the first attempt. Difficult intubations have been associated with pulmonary aspiration, and carry a high mortality rate in the obstetrical population. Every anaesthetist must have a plan for managing a failed intubation in the parturient. Persistent attempts without alterations in technique will only result in airway edema and trauma, with subsequent maternal and fetal hypoxemia. Serious hypoxemia can occur after 1 minute of apnea despite pre-oxygenation.

Maintaining cricoid pressure at all times is imperative. In the event of a failed intubation, gentle ventilation with 100% oxygen using the reservoir bag and mask may be all that is necessary until the patient awakes. When the parturient has recovered from the effects of the general anaesthetic agents, a regional technique or alternatively an 'awake intubation' with topical anaesthesia may be chosen. If there is fetal distress, the anaesthetist may decide to proceed with the anaesthetic using a volatile agent and ventilating the patient by bag and mask until she begins breathing spontaneously. If hypoxemia persists and attempts to ventilate the parturient are unsuccessful, a cricothyroidotomy with a large-bore needle and oxygen insufflation may be life-saving. Discuss with the staff anaesthesiologists what other options they would consider for managing this problem.

Induction of anaesthesia in the obstetrical patient may be accomplished by administering a reduced dose of thiopental, propofol, or ketamine (see induction agents, chapter 11). Muscle relaxation for intubation is provided using succinylcholine, while anaesthesia is maintained with 50% nitrous oxide and oxygen, and 0.5 MAC of a volatile agent such as isoflurane. Once the infant is delivered, narcotics and other agents may be used to deepen the level of anaesthesia.

Intermediate-acting muscle relaxants such as atracurium or vecuronium, when used, are reversed at the end of the procedure with a combination of anti-cholinesterase and anticholinergic agents (eg. edrophonium-atropine, or neostigmine-glycopyrrolate). The patient is ventilated with 100% oxygen. Extubation is performed after suctioning the upper airway secretions with the patient positioned on her side, and responding to verbal commands.

Notes:

Notes:

CHAPTER 19

Basic Neonatal Resuscitation

ROBERT CIRONE MD, AND ROBERT ELLIOT MD, FRCPC

Approximately six percent of newborn infants will require resuscitation of some kind in the delivery room. Health care workers providing care during labour and delivery should ensure that they have the knowledge and skills to resuscitate the newborn infant. Recently, major efforts have been made to provide delivery room care-givers with neonatal resuscitation guidelines through the Neonatal Resuscitation Program (NRP).

The purpose of this chapter is to introduce student's to the basic ABCs of neonatal resuscitation. We do not expect students to develop specific skills, such as intubation of the depressed neonate, or to use neonatal resuscitation drugs during their clerkship training. Nevertheless, we hope to stimulate their desire to develop neonatal resuscitation skills, and encourage them to attend a Neonatal Resuscitation Workshop and become a certified NRP provider.

Fetal Heart Rate (FHR) Monitoring:
Fetal heart rate monitoring is currently the most accurate screening technique for assessing fetal well being in-utero. Fetal heart rate monitoring can be done intermittently with a stethoscope, or continuously. Continuous monitoring is performed externally with either an abdominal electrocardiogram (ECG),

doppler ultrasound or phonocardiogram. It may also be done internally, by attaching an electrode to the fetal scalp when the head presents at the cervix during labour. Unlike intermittent monitoring, continuous monitoring facilitates the analysis of FHR trends, and their relation to uterine contractions.

What are the broad principles of neonatal resuscitation that I should know?*
1. Clear the airway.
2. Keep the infant warm and dry.
3. Provide physical Stimulation.
4. Assess the infants breathing and circulation.
5. Consider interventions.
   (oral suctioning, airway insertion, mask ventilation, intubation, endotracheal ventilation, external cardiac massage, fluid resuscitation, drug administration).

*What is the APGAR score**?*
The Apgar score is a clinical evaluation of the status of a newborn infant. It assigns a value of 0, 1, or 2 points to five variables, with the highest possible score being 10. It was devised by an American anesthesiologist, Dr. Virginia Apgar. The score is typically recorded 1 and 5 minutes after birth, however, one may continue to assess at 5 minute intervals in depressed infants requiring resuscitation. The most important vari-

Score	0	1	2
Heart Rate	Absent	< 100	> 100
Respiration	Absent	Slow, irregular	Good Crying
Colour	Blue, pale	Body pink, hands/feet blue	Completely Pink
Reflex Irritability	Absent	Grimace	Cough, sneeze
Muscle Tone	Limp	Some Flexion	Active Movement

Table 19.1: The Apgar Score **

able is the heart rate. An apgar score of ≤ 6 at five minutes correlates with increased morbidity and mortality. Resuscitation should never be postponed so that a "1-minute Apgar" can be done. The five variables measured can be recalled using the individual letters of Dr. Apgar's surname.

A = Appearance (Colour)
P = Pulse (Heart rate)
G = Grimace (Reflex irritability)
A = Activity (Muscle tone)
R = Respiration

What is asphyxia*?
Neonatal asphyxia is the combined result of a reduced oxygen supply, and an accumulation of carbon dioxide in the newborn infant. This may occur before, at the time of, or immediately following delivery. The need for more than *one minute of positive pressure ventilation* before sustained respirations are established, or an *Apgar score < 6 at five minutes*, is used in making a clinical diagnosis of asphyxia. The presence of perinatal asphyxia increases the infants risk of morbidity and mortality.

What is a normal FHR*?
The normal fetal heart rate in a term infant ranges from 120 to 160 beats per minute. It normally varies by 5 to 20 beats per minute. A premature infant (i.e., less than 37 weeks gestation) has an average FHR of 130 to 170 beats per minute, which is slightly higher than the term infant.

A fetal heart recording with a normal rate, but lacking variability, may be observed when the fetus is asleep, or premature. It may also occur when the infant has been exposed to drugs through the mother (narcotics, sedatives, anaesthetics, etc.), or from chronic fetal asphyxia. A completely "flat" baseline, (i.e. a FHR without variability) suggests either a previous insult that has been corrected, or ongoing congenital nervous and cardiac anomalies. The fetal heart normally increases in rate when the baby is active.

How are the fetal heart and lungs different from the adult?
In the fetal circulation, blood is able to pass from the right heart to the left heart through two channels which bypass the fetal lungs. The *ductus arteriosus* acts as a conduit for blood to

pass from the pulmonary artery directly to the aorta. The *foramen ovale* allows blood from the right atrium to pass directly to the left atrium. The amount of pulmonary arterial blood flowing through the fetal lungs is small due to their small volume and high vascular resistance. Blood from the right ventricle bypasses the lungs and eventually flows through the low resistance placenta where it picks up maternal oxygen and excretes waste products of metabolism (carbon dioxide, urea, etc.) see figure 19.1.

The fetal lungs contain an ultrafiltrate of plasma equivalent to their functional residual capacity (FRC) volume of about 30 ml/kg. During vaginal delivery, most of this fluid is "squeezed" out of the lungs, facilitating initial lung expansion and oxygen exchange. Infants born by caesarean section do not have this "squeeze" and may have more fluid in their lungs, impairing lung expansion, and oxygenation. This condition is frequently termed transient tachypnea of the newborn, and may require supplemental oxygen therapy and observation for the first 24 hours.

Why do infants breathe when they are born?

When the umbilical cord is clamped, the low resistance placenta is removed from the infants circulation. The result is an increase in the vascular resistance in the aorta, left ventricle, and left atrium associated with a rise in left sided pressures. This creates a functional closure of the foramen ovale and the ductus arteriosus. As these right to left shunt paths are closed, blood is diverted into the lungs. A combination of mild acidosis, hypoxia, touch, noise, pain, and cold all stimulate the infant to take their first breath. The vaginal squeeze referred to above, facilitates lung expansion. Fresh oxygen in the alveoli and the expanded lung volume decrease the resistance to blood flowing into the lungs.

Hypoxia, cold, acidosis, hypovolemia, hypoventilation, hypercarbia, and atelectasis will all increase pulmonary vascular resistance, forcing blood through the foramen ovale and ductus arteriosus. These factors tend to cause a *persistent fetal circulation* and impede

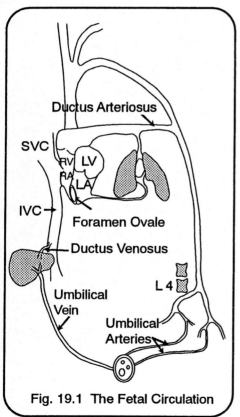

Fig. 19.1 The Fetal Circulation

the newborns oxygenation and ventilation.

What fetal heart rate patterns should I be concerned about*?
FHR *decelerations* may indicate a change in the baby's well-being in utero and are most significant if the rate drops below 100 bpm. *Early* decelerations occurring with contractions and then returning to baseline are probably a reflex response to head compression during the contraction and are usually benign. *Late* decelerations are more ominous, usually occurring with contractions and having a delayed return to the baseline FHR. They often signify fetal hypoxia and acidosis. *Variable* decelerations are not associated with contractions, have a quick onset and recovery. They are due to transient cord compression, and are usually benign. *Sustained bradycardia* with a FHR < 100, indicates serious fetal distress, and requires urgent intervention. Sustained tachycardia is often associated with fever or sepsis, but may be observed as a response to maternal drug administration (e.g., atropine or ephedrine).

If serious FHR decelerations occur, what can I do*?
Ensure adequate left uterine displacement to *prevent aortocaval compression* (see chapter 18: Obstetrical Anaesthesia). *Provide supplemental oxygen* to the mother. A common way of administering oxygen is by fitting a face mask with rebreathing reservoir bag on the mother and setting the oxygen flow rate to ≥ 6 litres per minute. *Discontinue the oxytocin* infusion if it is being ad-

ministered. Consider changing maternal positions for variable decelerations. Evaluate and *correct any maternal hypotension* using an intravenous fluid bolus and/or ephedrine. Summon help. *Ensure accurate FHR monitoring,* rule out artifacts and consider more intensive fetal monitoring such as a fetal scalp clip for continuous internal FHR monitoring.

What is meconium*?
Meconium refers to the first discharge from the infants intestinal tract. It has a green appearance and consists of epithelial cells, mucus, and bile. When meconium is passed by the infant in utero, it colours the amniotic fluid and indicates that the infant has been subjected to a stress at some time. Meconium excretion in utero is observed more frequently in the term or post term infant. A thick "pea-soup" meconium may suggest a recent episode of hypoxia and prompt more aggressive fetal monitoring or management of the labour and delivery.

Infants that inhale meconium into their trachea and lungs may have difficulty with oxygenation, ventilation and may develop complications such as a pneumothorax or pneumonitis. Meconium may collect in the pharynx in the infant and may be inhaled into the lungs with their first breath. It is paramount that these infants have *thorough suctioning of their mouth, pharynx, and nasopharynx at the time the head is delivered* and prior to their first breath with delivery of the chest. The clinician may also decide to intubate the infant immediately after delivery to

---

Risk Factors

Antepartum

- Age > 35
- Diabetes
- Pregnancy induced hypertension.
- Chronic hypertension.
- No Prenatal Care.
- Maternal Substance abuse.
- Rh sensitization.
- Drug therapy (Mg, Li, adrenergic drugs, etc.)
- Other CVS, Neuro, or Thyroid illness.
- Previous stillbirth.
- 2nd or 3rd trimester bleeding
- Hydramnios
- Oligohydramnios
- Multiple gestation.
- Post-term.
- Small for dates.
- Fetal malformation.

Intrapartum

- Abnormal presentation.
- Operative delivery.
- Premature labour.
- Premature rupture of membranes.
- Precipitous labour.
- Prolonged labour.
- FHR abnormalities.
- Maternal narcotics (within 4 hrs. of delivery).
- General anaesthesia.
- Meconium stained fluid.
- Prolapsed cord.
- Placental abruption.
- Placenta previa.
- Uterine tetany.

Table 19.2: Risk Factors predicting the need for neonatal resuscitation.

---

suction as much meconium from the trachea as possible.

Can I predict which infant may need resuscitation at delivery?
Infants requiring resuscitation may have associated pre-existing maternal risk factors, complications arising during labour and delivery, or underlying fetal risk factors. (Risk factors associated with the need for neonatal resuscitation are presented in table 19.2 for reference purpose only).

How do I make sure that I am ready to provide resuscitation for the newborn infant?
1. At every delivery, at least one indi-vidual should be capable of perform-ing a complete resuscitation (i.e., including endotracheal intubation and the use of medications). In many cases, this is the person delivering the infant.

2. Even for cases when a normal infant is expected, a second person who will be primarily responsible for the infant, must be present in the delivery room. This person must be able to initiate a resuscitation and assist the fully trained person, should a full resuscitation become necessary.

3. When neonatal asphyxia is antici-pated, two individuals whose sole responsibility is to the infant, should be present in the delivery room and

be prepared to work as a team to perform a complete resuscitation. The person delivering the infant should not be counted as one of the two resuscitators.

4. With multiple births, a team is needed for each infant.

5. There should be no delay in initiating resuscitation; waiting a few minutes for someone "on-call" to arrive is an unacceptable practice and invites disaster.

Radiant heater
Stethoscope
Suction and suction catheters
Oxygen source and tubing
Neonatal resuscitation.bag
Airway pressure manometer
Face masks, Oral airways.
Endotracheal tubes (2.5, 3, 3.5)
ETT Stylet
Laryngoscope
Straight blades No. 0 & 1
Medications (see text)
Umbilical catheters (3.5 and 5 Fr.)
Umbilical catheter tray
Needles and syringes
ECG monitor

Table 19.3: Basic Neonatal Resuscitation Equipment.

Equipment: (see table 19.3)
(for reference only).

1. Equipment and medications should be checked daily, and prior to anticipated use.

2. The delivery room should be kept relatively warm and the radiant heater should be preheated. Warm blankets can also be helpful in preventing excessive heat loss from the neonate.

The Basics:

I: Open the Airway.**

• Position the infant supine or on their side with the neck either in a neutral position or slightly extended. Avoid overextension or flexion, which may produce airway obstruction. A slight trendelenburg position is also helpful.

• A 1" folded towel under the infants shoulders may be useful if the infant has a large occiput.

• If the infant has absent, slow, or difficult respirations, apply suction first to the *mouth and then nose.* If the nose is cleared first, the infant may gasp and aspirate secretions in the pharynx. If mechanical suctioning with an 8F or 10F catheter is used, make sure the vacuum does not exceed -100 mm Hg. Limit suctioning to 5 seconds at a time and *monitor heart rate for bradycardia,* which may occur with deep oropharyngeal stimulation.

• If meconium is present in the amniotic fluid, special endotracheal suctioning may be required in the depressed infant.

II: Keep the infant warm and dry.**

Place the infant under an overhead radiant heater. Dry the body and head to remove amniotic fluid and prevent heat loss. The gentle stimulation will also help initiate and maintain breathing.

III: Physical Stimulation.

- If drying and suctioning do not induce effective breathing, gently slapping or flicking the soles of the feet or rubbing the infants back may be useful.
- Do not waste time continuing tactile stimulation if there is no response after 10 - 15 seconds.

IV: Evaluate the infant.

Respirations: Infants who are apneic or gasping despite brief stimulation attempts should receive positive pressure ventilation.

Heart Rate: Monitor either by auscultating the apical beat or by palpating the base of the umbilical cord. If the heart rate is below 100 bpm, begin positive-pressure ventilation, even if the infant is making some respiratory efforts.

Colour: The presence of central cyanosis indicates that although there is enough oxygen passing through the lungs to maintain the heart rate, the infant is still not well oxygenated. A face mask with oxygen at 5 L/min. should be held closely to the infants face until the infant becomes pink.

Technique of Positive Pressure Ventilation (PPV):

Ventilatory support is required when**:

- Apnea or gasping respirations are present.
- The heart rate is less than 100 bpm.
- Central cyanosis persists despite 100% oxygen.

Most neonates can be adequately ventilated with a bag and mask (see figure 19.3). The assisted **ventilatory rate** should be between **40 - 60 breaths per minute.** Initial lung inflation pressures may be as high as 30 - 40 cm of H_2O to

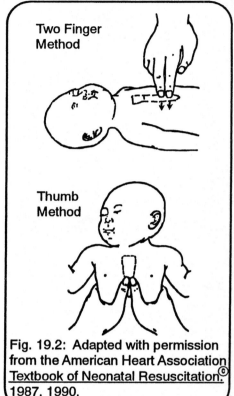

Fig. 19.2: Adapted with permission from the American Heart Association Textbook of Neonatal Resuscitation.[C] 1987, 1990.

overcome the elastic forces of the lungs if the infant has not taken their first breath. Subsequent ventilation should be achieved with airway pressures of 15 -20 cm H_2O.

Adequate ventilation is assessed by** observing chest wall motion and hearing breath sounds bilaterally. If chest expansion is inadequate:

- reposition the head; consider extending the head a bit further and repositioning the shoulder towel.
- suction any secretions.
- consider an oral airway, and ventilating with the infants mouth slightly open.
- increase ventilation pressures to 20 - 40 cm H_2O
- if unsuccessful, abandon the bag and mask technique, and intubate.

After 15 - 30 seconds of effective ventilation, the heart rate of the neonate should be re-evaluated. The heart rate over a 6 second period is counted and multiplied by 10 to give an approximation of the 1-minute heart rate. (e.g., 8 beats in 6 seconds = 80 bpm).

Positive pressure ventilation can be gradually withdrawn if the HR > 100 and spontaneous breathing efforts are present. The care provider should continue to provide physical stimulation and supplemental O_2 to the infant.

If the HR is less than 100, ventilation should continue. Chest compressions are initiated if the HR is less than 80 and decreasing. When the heart rate is less than 60, immediate ventilation with 100% oxygen is instituted with simultaneous chest compressions.

Chest Compressions:
Compression of the sternum results in compression of the heart and increases intrathoracic pressure. During compression, blood is pumped into the arterial circulation. Release of the sternum results in an increase in venous return to the heart. Chest compressions must be

accompanied by ventilation with 100% oxygen. Asphyxia in the neonate not only slows the heart rate but decreases myocardial contractility, resulting in diminished blood flow and oxygen delivery to vital organs.

When should I start chest compressions**?
You should begin chest compressions when the heart rate remains below 80 bpm despite PPV with 100% O_2. Chest compressions can be discontinued when the heart rate is 80 bpm or greater.

What is the proper technique for administering chest compressions to an infant**?
There are two methods of compressing the chest in infants. Using the *thumb method*, both hands encircle the torso, with the fingers supporting the back, while the thumbs are positioned side by side over the sternum, creating chest compression with downward displacement of the sternum. Using the *two-finger approach*, the middle and ring fingers of one hand are held perpendicular to the chest as the finger tips apply pressure to the sternum. The other hand is used to support the infants back from below (see figure 19.2).
The amount of pressure applied with compressions is adjusted to achieve *1.5 cm of displacement*. A full "cycle" consists of both a compression and release phase. This rate is adjusted to achieve 2 cycles per second or *120 compressions per minute*.

Once the fingers (thumbs) have been correctly positioned over the sternum, care should be taken to ensure that the hands are not moved from this position. Valuable time may be wasted attempting to relocate the correct hand position. Complications of incorrect hand placement and chest compression include fractured ribs, lacerated spleen, and pneumothorax.

When the infant is *intubated* and receiving simultaneous ventilation and chest compressions, ventilation at a rate of 40 - 60 per minute with independent, concurrent chest compressions at a rate of 120 per minute is recommended.

Air may be forced into the infants stomach if they are receiving simultaneous PPV (with a bag and mask) and chest compressions. Hence when the infant is being ventilated with a *bag and mask,* ventilation should be interposed between compressions. Every three chest compressions are followed by a pause to interpose an effective breath. The resulting 90 compressions with 30 ventilations yield a combined rate of compressions and ventilation of 120 per minute. The variation in recommended rates of ventilation and chest compressions between the intubated and non intubated infant is an attempt to minimize the risk of gastric distention and (or) aspiration.

Compressions are interrupted after the first 30 seconds, to make a six second heart rate count. Compressions are stopped once the heart rate is above 80, and ventilation is stopped when the heart rate is above 100.

Endotracheal intubation is indicated when*:

- Prolonged PPV is required (to minimize gastric distention).
- Ventilation with a bag and mask is ineffective (poor chest expansion, persistent low HR).
- Tracheal suctioning required (thick or particulate meconium).
- Diaphragmatic hernia suspected (to prevent bowel distension in the chest).

While endotracheal intubation may play an essential part of an infants resuscitation, it is neither the purpose, nor in the scope of this chapter to discuss the technique, confirmation, or complications of this intervention. We hope that this chapter will provide you with a stepping stone for your future courses in neonatal resuscitation.

*Which four common drugs used in resuscitation of the depressed neonate should I be familiar with?***

1. Oxygen.
2. Intravenous Fluids.
3. Epinephrine.
4. Naloxone.

Oxygen:

For the majority of infants who require resuscitation, the only medication needed will be 100% oxygen delivered with effective ventilation. Some will require chest compressions, and a small minority of resuscitated infants will require other medications, such as epinephrine, intravenous fluid resuscitation, or other special drugs.

Intravenous fluids:
How will I know whether or not the infant is hypovolemic?

Conditions which result in acute maternal hypovolemia prior to delivery of the infant, should make the clinician suspicious that the infant may also be suffering from the effects of hypovolemia. Maternal hemorrhage prior to delivery is one such condition. A few of the causes of maternal hemorrhage prior to delivery include placental abruption, placenta previa, transection of the placenta during caesarean section, and maternal trauma. Other conditions that may result in neonatal hypovolemia include multiple gestation pregnancies, umbilical cord tear during delivery, and a strangulating umbilical cord requiring umbilical cord transection for delivery.

Hypovolemia occurs more frequently in the newborn than is commonly recognized. Blood loss is often not obvious and initial tests of hemoglobin and hematocrit are usually misleading. The increase in vascular volume secondary to a volume expander should improve tissue perfusion and reduce the development of metabolic acidosis.

Clinical signs of hypovolemia resulting from an acute loss of greater than 20% of the blood volume include:
• Pallor persisting after oxygenation.
• A weak pulse despite a good heart rate.
• A poor response to resuscitative efforts.
• A decreased blood pressure (< 55/30).

What is the normal blood pressure and blood volume in a term infant?

On average, the blood pressure in a term infant is 70/44. Hypotension in the neonate has been defined as a systolic blood pressure of less than 50 mm Hg in a term infant (see table 19.4). The normal blood volume in a term neonate is 80 - 100 ml/kg. Hence in a 3 kg infant with a blood volume of 250 ml, a loss of only 50 ml represents 20% of their blood volume.

Weight (grams)	SBP	DBP	MAP
1000-2000	49	26	35
2000-3000	59	32	43
>3000	70	44	53

Table 19.4: Average blood pressures at birth.

What conditions, other than hypovolemia, may result in hypotension in the neonate?
Other conditions include:
• Hypoglycaemia (diabetic mother)
• Hypocalcemia (Intrauterine asphyxia)
• Hypermagnesemia (Mg^{2+} therapy for the pre-eclamptic mother)
• Sepsis (chorioamnionitis or prolonged rupture of membranes)
• Pneumothorax (meconium aspiration)
• Cardiac pathology
• Diaphragmatic hernia

Assuming we've made a correct diagnosis of hypovolemia, how can we correct it?
The most commonly used volume expanders are normal saline and ringer's lactate. Other volume expanders include 5% albumen, and O-negative blood cross matched with the mother's blood. The volume of fluid administered should be equivalent to 10 ml/kg, and this should be given as an infusion over 5 - 10 minutes. In a 3 kg infant this would be equivalent to 30 ml.

Epinephrine:

When should I consider giving epinephrine*?
Epinephrine is indicated if no heart rate can be detected or if the heart rate persists below 80 bpm despite adequate ventilation with 100% oxygen and chest compressions for at least 30 seconds.

Why is epinephrine such an important drug in neonatal resuscitation?
Epinephrine has both α (alpha) and β (beta) adrenergic stimulating properties. The alpha effect causes vasoconstriction which raises the perfusion pressure during chest compressions, augmenting oxygen delivery to both the heart and brain. The beta effect enhances cardiac contractility, stimulates spontaneous contractions and increases the heart rate.

How can I give epinephrine?
Epinephrine can be given either intravenously or by the endotracheal tube every 3 to 5 minutes as required. The epinephrine concentration used in neonatal resuscitation is supplied as a *1:10,000* dilution (i.e. 1 gram in 10,000

ml or 0.1 mg per ml). The intravenous dose is 0.01 to 0.03 mg per kg. In a 3 kg infant, a *1/4 ml to 3/4 ml of epinephrine* would be an appropriate starting dose, as this would be equivalent to 25 to 75 mcg (approximately 0.01 to 0.03 mg/kg). If an intravenous route is unavailable, epinephrine can be given through the endotracheal tube. Epinephrine given by endotracheal route should be diluted with 1-2 ml of saline. When given by the ETT, plasma concentrations may be lower compared to the intravenous route. If the infant does not respond to the initial ETT epinephrine dose, the endotracheal epinephrine dose is increased by a factor of ten (0.1 - 0.2 mg/kg).

Naloxone*:
What is naloxone and when should I consider giving it?
Naloxone is a pure opioid antagonist without intrinsic respiratory depression activity. Naloxone is indicated for the reversal of respiratory depression when the mother has received opioids within 4 hours of delivery and the infant is observed to have depressed respirations. While naloxone works very rapidly, adequate ventilatory assistance should always be provided first. The duration of naloxone is shorter than that of some opioids, making respiratory monitoring mandatory for a further 4 to 6 hours.

Naloxone can be given either intravenously or by an endotracheal tube. Subcutaneous or intramuscular routes can also be used if the infants perfusion is adequate, however, the onset of action may be slower with these routes. If maternal opioid addiction is suspect-

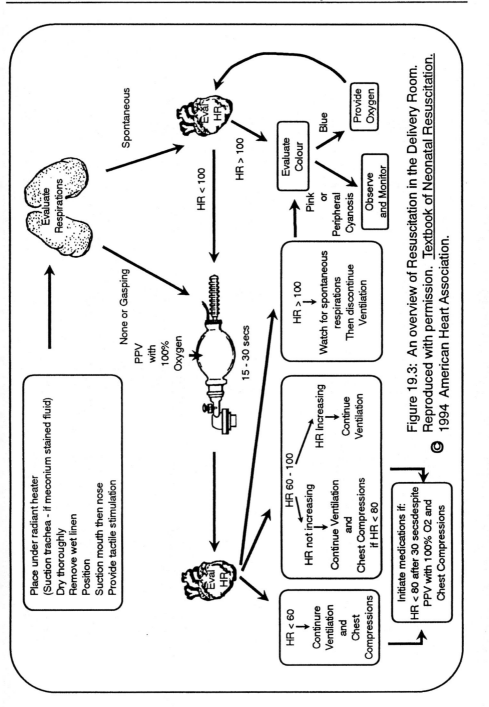

Figure 19.3: An overview of Resuscitation in the Delivery Room. Reproduced with permission. Textbook of Neonatal Resuscitation. © 1994 American Heart Association.

ed, it is probably prudent not to give naloxone. Rather, simply support ventilation until respiratory drive is adequate. Administrating naloxone to infants of opioid dependent mothers may result is a withdrawal reaction and severe seizures in the infant. Naloxone is supplied in a 0.4 mg/ml concentration for neonatal resuscitation. The dose is 0.1 mg/kg for infant resuscitation, and hence a typical 3 kg infant would require *3/4 of a ml* (iv, ETT, im, or sc) of naloxone (0.4 mg/ml) as an initial dose.

Notes:

References:

1. Bloom RS, Cropley C. Textbook of Neonatal Resuscitation. ed. Chameides L and the AHA/AHP Neonatal Resuscitation Steering Committee. American Heart Association, 1990.

2. Emergency Cardiac Care Committee and Subcommittees, American Heart Association. Guidelines for cardiopulmonary resuscitation and emergency cardiac care, VII: neonatal resuscitation. JAMA 1992; 268:2276-2281.

3. Christenson JM, Solimano AJ, Williams J, et al. The new American Heart Association guidelines for cardiopulmonary resuscitation and emergency care: presented by the Emergency Cardiac Care Subcommittee of the Heart and Stoke Foundation of Canada. Can Med Assoc J 1993;149:585-590.

Notes:

CHAPTER 20

Intravenous Fluid and Blood Component Therapy

WAYNE BARRY MD., FRCPC

Optimal perioperative fluid therapy requires an understanding of the changes that occur in the volume and composition of the body fluid compartments. Intravenous fluids are used to replenish fluid losses while maintaining the blood volume, coagulation status, and oxygen delivery. Inadequate fluid therapy risks organ hypoperfusion, coagulopathy, and electrolyte imbalances. Excessive fluid therapy risks circulatory overload as well as organ and tissue edema. To avoid inadequate or excessive fluid therapy, the clinician must makes serial evaluations of the patients fluid requirements in terms of their *maintenance fluids, fluid deficit, third space losses, and ongoing blood losses.*

With this in mind, this chapter shall enable the reader to calculate:

1. *Maintenance* fluid requirements
2. Fluid *deficit* estimation
3. Ongoing fluid *3rd space* losses, and
4. Fluids required to replace *blood* lost.

We shall also review the indications and complications of transfusing blood products.

Body Fluid Compartments:
Total body water (TBW) constitutes 60% of the body weight, or approximately 42 liters in a 70 kg adult. Two thirds of the TBW is contained within cells as intracellular fluid (ICF). The ICF represents 40% of the body weight, which is approximately 28 liters in a 70 kg adult. The remaining 1/3 of the TBW exists outside the cells as extracellular fluid (ECF). It represents 20% of the body weight or 14 liters of water in a 70 kg adult (see table 20.1).

Sodium (140 meq/l) and potassium (150 meq/l) are the principle cations in the ECF and ICF respectively. Albumen (40 gm/l) is the primary molecule responsible for the oncotic pressure generated by the ECF. Aldosterone and antidiuretic hormone (ADH) increase the extracellular fluid volume by increasing salt (aldosterone) and water (ADH) reabsorption. Atrial natriuretic protein decreases the ECF volume by promoting salt and water excretion.

I. Maintenance Fluid Requirements*:
Intravenous fluid requirements for periods of less than one week can be provided for with water, sodium, and

Compartment	% Body Weight	Volume in liters / 70 kg
Total		
Male (70 kg)	60	42
Female (70 kg)	50	35
ECF[†]	20	14
Plasma	4	2.8
Interstitial Fluid	16	11.2
ICF	40	28

Table 20.1: Distribution of body water. [†]The ECF represents approximately 1/3 (range 27 - 45%) of the total body mass, while the ICF occupies approximately 2/3 of the total body mass.

potassium. Chloride, magnesium, calcium, and other trace mineral supplementation is required for patients needing chronic intravenous maintenance therapy. As hyperglycemia is a normal response to surgery, dextrose is recommended only for those patients at risk of hypoglycemia (e.g., infants and diabetic patients).

A normal 70 kg adult requires approximately 2.5 liters of water a day with 75 meq of sodium, and 40 meq of potassium. Water and salt administration in excess of this, will result in their excretion in the urine (provided cardiac and renal function are normal).

Intravenous fluids for a period of > 24 hours and < 1 week: Preoperative fluid requirements during this period of time can usually be met with a solution of 2/3 of 5% dextrose with 1/3 normal saline (referred to as 2/3rds, 1/3rd) with 15 - 20 meq of potassium per liter. Alternatively, we could use a solution

of 1/2 normal saline with 15 - 20 meq of potassium per liter. At maintenance infusion rates, this will meet the patients daily water, sodium and potassium requirements.

Intravenous fluids for surgery scheduled to be performed within 24 hours: Normal saline, or ringer's lactate are the preoperative intravenous fluids of choice for surgery scheduled within 24 hours. The rationale for this recommendation includes:

1. Potassium replacement is not required for brief periods of time.

2. Intravenous fluids containing potassium pose a potential hazard should the patient receive an inadvertent fluid bolus (e.g., rapid i.v. administration for hypotension associated with the induction of anaesthesia).

3. Normal saline and ringer's lactate are the most common fluids administered intraoperatively, as they are used to replenish the sodium rich plasma and interstitial fluid compartments.

Table 20.2:	Maintenance water requirements	
	Per hour**	Per Day**
1st to 10th kg	4 ml/kg	100 ml/kg
11th to 20th kg	2 ml/kg	50 ml/kg
21st to nth kg	1 ml/kg	20 ml/kg

Exercise caution when administering crystalloids such as NS or RL to patients with congestive heart failure, renal failure, or advanced age. In these patients, a preoperative intravenous solution of 2/3rds and 1/3rd may be more appropriate.

Maintenance fluid requirements for any body weight can be calculated using the "4-2-1" rule for hourly fluid requirements or the "100-50-20" rule for daily fluid requirements (see table 20.2). For example, a 75 kg adult will require:

Per hour:

	10 kg x 4 ml/hr = 40 ml/hr
	10 kg x 2 ml/hr = 20 ml/hr
	55 kg x 1 ml/hr = 55 ml/hr
Total:	75 kg 115 ml/hr

Per day:

	10 kg x 100 ml/day = 1000 ml
	10 kg x 50 ml/day = 500 ml
	55 kg x 20 ml/day = 1100 ml
Total: 75 kg	2600 ml/day

II: Fluid Deficit Estimation*:
A fluid deficit may develop as a result of a period of fasting or a pathologic process. The fluid deficit from fasting can be calculated by multiplying the patient's hourly maintenance require-ments by the number of hours fasted. (Fluid Deficit = Maintenance requirements per hour x number of hours fasted). A fluid deficit resulting from a pathological process is much more difficult to quantify accurately. Table 20.3 lists clinical conditions frequently associated with fluid deficits, with associated physical and laboratory findings. For example, a patient with a fractured hip may have 1 - 2 liters of blood sequestered in their thigh tissues. When such significant fluid deficits are not appreciated and corrected prior to anaesthesia, profound cardiovascular collapse may occur with induction of anaesthesia.

III. Third Space Losses*:
A reduction in ECF volume during surgery results from evaporative losses, exudative losses, tissue edema secondary to surgical manipulation, and fluid sequestration in organs, such as the bowel and lung. These fluid losses can be surprisingly extensive. The simplest guideline for replacing third space fluid losses is a *4 - 6 - 8 ml/kg/hr* rule. Four for minor, 6 for moderate, and 8 ml/kg/hr for major surgical trauma. For example, we can anticipate that a bowel resection will have 6 ml/kg/hr of 3rd space fluid losses during the operation. This fluid is usually administered as

Table 20.3: Common conditions associated with preoperative fluid deficits.	
• Fractured hip, femur, pelvis • Bowel obstruction • Preoperative bowel preparation • Trauma	• Protracted vomiting and diarrhea • Burns • Sepsis • Pancreatitis
Common physical findings supporting a preoperative fluid deficit.	
• Tachycardia • Orthostatic hypotension • Supine hypotension • Oliguria (< 0.5 ml/kg/hr)	• Tachypnea • Decreased jugular venous pressure (JVP) • Dry mucous membranes • Decreased tissue turgor
Common laboratory findings associated with a fluid deficit.	
• Elevated urea • Elevated creatinine • Low urinary sodium concentration (U_{Na} < 20 mM)	• Elevated urine osmolarity • Elevated hematocrit

either normal saline or ringer's lactate, and must be given in addition to the patient's maintenance requirements, calculated fluid deficit, and ongoing blood losses. Mobilization of third space fluid occurs approximately 72 hours after surgery, and may result in circulatory overload in the patient with compromised cardiac or renal function.

IV. Blood Loss Replacement*:
Intravenous *crystalloid or colloid* solutions may be administered to replenish the intravascular volume. Crystalloid solutions are salt containing solutions that are semipermeable to cellular membranes. Examples of crystalloid solutions include NS, RL, and 2/3, 1/3 intravenous solutions. By contrast, colloid intravenous solutions contain aggregates of molecules that resist diffusion across cellular membranes. Colloid

solutions may be synthetic (e.g., pentaspan, hetaspan, dextran), or collected from the donor blood pool (eg. albumen, plasma, whole blood).

If 1000 ml of NS is infused intravenously, only 1/3 (approx. 300 ml) will remain in the intravascular compartment. The remaining 2/3 (~ 700 ml) will move into the interstitial and intracellular compartments. As a consequence, 3 to 5 times the volume of blood lost must be infused when crystalloids such as NS or RL are used to maintain the intravascular volume. With colloid solutions, however, blood losses can be replaced on a 1:1 volume basis.

D5W:
Similarly, the intravenous administration of 1000 ml of D5W (5% dextrose in

Table 20.4:		Common intravenous solutions and their components.						
Solution	Dextrose gm/dl	Na	Cl	K	pH	Osm	Other	
			meq/l					
Plasma		140	103	4	7.4	290	Ca 5 meq/l	
D5W	5				5.0	253		
2/3 D5W,1/3 NS	3.3	51	51		4.8	270		
2/3,1/3 + 20 meq KCL	3.3	51	51	20	4.8	290		
0.9% Saline (NS)		154	154		5.7	308		
Ringer's lactate		130	109	4	6.7	273	Ca 1.5meq/l, lactate 20 meq/l	
0.45% Saline (½NS)		77	77		5.3	154		
Pentaspan		154	154		5.0	326	10 gm/dl pentastarch	

water), results in minimal intravascular volume expansion, because most of the fluid moves into the interstitial and intracellular compartments. Hyponatremia, hyperglycemia and a decrease in serum osmolarity will result when large volumes of D5W are infused. For these reasons, D5W is a poor choice for correcting a blood volume deficit. Moreover, large amounts of D5W should be avoided in patients receiving oxytocin, because oxytocin's inherent ADH effect may result in hyponatremia and water intoxication.

The severity of an ischemic cerebral event may be increased if iatrogenic hyperglycemia is induced with the administration of dextrose containing fluids. This has special relevance for neurosurgical procedures, and patients with cerebrovascular pathology.

Saline:
The infusion of large amounts of intravenous NS (e.g., trauma resuscitation) may be accompanied with a hyperchloremic, hypernatremic non anion gap metabolic acidosis. In trauma patients, this source of acidosis is commonly overlooked by clinicians. An increase in minute ventilation, produces a respiratory alkalosis, which is the normal compensation for an acute metabolic acidosis. This additional respiratory work, in a spontaneously breathing patient, may be detrimental in a patient with other coexisting disease.

Chronic gastric losses may produce a hypochloremic metabolic alkalosis. The administration of NS can be used to correct this abnormality.

Ringer's lactate:

Ringer's lactate solution contains 4 meq/l of potassium, and should be used with caution in patients with pre-existing hyperkalemia or renal failure. Patients with chronic diarrhea may develop a hyperchloremic metabolic acidosis. This will respond to treatment with a bicarbonate (lactate) containing solution, such as ringer's lactate.

The administration of hypotonic solutions to patients with brain injury may contribute to brain cell swelling. As saline is relatively more hypertonic than RL, it is generally the preferred crystalloid for these patients (see table 20.4).

Pentaspan:

Pentaspan has the same sodium and chloride concentration as NS. Each 100 ml contains an additional 10 grams of pentastarch, of which 70% is eliminated by the kidneys within 24 hours. The plasma volume expansion achieved is equal to the volume of pentaspan administered (1:1 ratio). Pentaspan is more expensive than crystalloid solutions, but less expensive than other blood substitutes such as albumen.

Note, however, that pentaspan is not a RBC substitute and has no oxygen carrying capacity. The hemodynamic effects of pentaspan are equal or superior to those of albumen. Both result in expansion of the plasma volume, with increases in preload, cardiac output, and oxygen delivery. Increases in bleeding and clotting times resulting from an infusion of albumen or pentastarch are believed to be secondary to a dilution of platelets and coagulation factors[4]. A maximum volume of 2000 ml per 24 hours is recommended.

Side effects of pentaspan include circulatory overload (pulmonary edema, congestive heart failure), altered coagulation (prolonged clotting times, prolonged INR and PTT), and hypersensitivity reactions such as wheezing and urticaria. It is contraindicated in patients with bleeding disorders, renal disease, and circulatory overload. It is supplied in 100, 250, and 500 ml infusion bags. Hetaspan and dextran are two other synthetic intravenous colloids. We use them less frequently at our centre because there is an increased incidence of anaphylactoid reactions associated with them.

Albumen:

Albumen is available as a 5% and 25% solution. It is heat treated at 60°C for 10 hours to eliminate bacterial and viral contamination. Administration of the 5% solution will produce an equal increase in intravascular volume expansion. Administration of the 25% solution will draw interstitial fluid into the intravascular space and increase the intravascular volume by a factor of 4 times the albumen volume. Albumen can be used as a plasma volume expander in patients with adequate oxygen carrying capacity, however it is not recommended as a method of correcting nutritional deficiencies.

Autologous blood:

Autologous blood involves the preoperative collection of blood from a patient who is scheduled to have surgery, and for whom one anticipates the need for a perioperative blood transfusion. Contrary to popular belief, autologous blood is discarded if it is not administered to the donor. As it is not placed in the general donor homologous blood pool, patients should not be encouraged to donate autologous blood on the basis that it could benefit someone else. Patients with bacterial or viral infections are not suitable donors, as there is a risk of exposing other patients to the contaminated blood (e.g., clerical error). Suitable candidates are able to donate a maximum of 1 unit of blood every 4 to 7 days, and should stop donating three or more days prior to the planned procedure. Unsuitable candidates include patients with a hemoglobin level less than 110 gm/L, and patients with unstable angina or critical aortic stenosis. As the maximum shelf life of stored blood is 35 days, a donor could donate up to 4 units prior to surgery. Oral iron and/or recombinant erythropoietin therapy may be used to increase the number of units that can be collected preoperatively. Autologous blood is not separated into components like homologous blood, but rather is stored as whole blood.

Acceptable blood loss*:

We do not have a universal answer to the question "What is the minimal acceptable hemoglobin?" Evidence suggests that a normal circulating blood volume can be reduced by as much as 25% with little stress being placed on the patient, provided that the intravascular blood volume is maintained. Animals are able to tolerate acute reductions in hemoglobin to levels between 30 to 50 gm/L. Such an acute decrease in hemoglobin is only tolerated when normovolemia is maintained, and mechanisms to increase oxygen transport by increasing cardiac output and 2,3 DPG levels are intact. Patients with cardiac disease or atherosclerotic lesions that restrict blood flow to vital organs are limited in their ability to adapt to acute anemia. A balance between the risk of transmitting an infectious disease, and the need for administering blood products for their oxygen carrying capacity and coagulation properties, must be reached in each patient undergoing surgery.

Postoperative hemoglobins in the range of 60 to 80 gm/L are now considered acceptable in patients who do not have cardiovascular disease. Transfusion should be used only to replace losses beyond this level. Nevertheless, even a modest anemia with hemoglobin levels of 80 to 100 gm/L requires an increase in heart rate and stroke volume to meet the body's oxygen requirements. This introduces an additional cardiac stress. Physicians must consider the consequences of this imposed cardiac stress when deciding to transfuse patients with moderate anemia and coexisting atherosclerosis or cardiovascular disease. In the end, each patient must be evaluated individually.

Questions that may be helpful in formulating a decision to administer blood products to a particular patient include:

1. Does the patient accept the possibility of receiving blood products?
2. If anemic, is this an acute anemia or

a chronic anemia to which the patient has adapted?

3. Is the patient likely to lose more blood in the immediate future?
4. Does the patient have risk factors for atherosclerosis, coronary artery disease, or cerebrovascular disease? (e.g., Smoking history, hypertension, diabetes, hypercholesterolemia, personal or family history of heart disease).
5. Is their evidence of a coagulopathy in which additional blood loss is anticipated (prolonged INR, PTT, or decreased platelets)?
6. Does the blood loss exceed what was calculated as the acceptable blood loss for this patient? (see text below).
7. Is the patient hemodynamically unstable despite other fluid resuscitation?

Table 20. 5	Blood Volume ml/kg
Premature infant	90
Term infant	80
Slim male	75
Obese male	70
Slim female	65
Obese female	60

Calculation of the acceptable blood loss:

Since, an adult male has a blood volume of 70 ml/kg (see table 20.5), the estimated blood volume (EBV) is 70 kg x 70 ml/kg = 4900 ml. If the initial hemoglobin is 150 gm/dl and we have decided that we will allow the hemoglobin to drop to 90 gm/L before trans-fusing blood products, we can calculate the acceptable blood loss (ABL).

$$ABL = \frac{Hb(i) - Hb(f)}{Hb(i.)} \times EBV$$

$Hb(i) =$ Initial hemoglobin $= 150$ gm/L

$Hb(f) =$ Final hemoglobin $= 90$ gm/L

Therefore:

$$ABL = \frac{150 - 90}{150} \times 4900 = 1960 \text{ ml}$$

The most common blood products administered are whole blood (autologous blood donors), packed red blood cells (RBCs), platelets, and fresh frozen plasma. One unit of whole blood has a volume of 500 ml, while a unit of packed RBCs has a volume of approximately 300 ml (including their anticoagulant volume). One unit of packed RBCs will raise the hemoglobin by 10 gm/L in the average adult. Alternatively, 3 ml/kg of RBCs will raise the hemoglobin by 10 gm/L. This later formula is useful for calculating the volume of blood required for transfusion in neonates and infants. Packed RBCs are indicated when there is a deficiency in the patients oxygen carrying capacity.

Fresh Frozen Plasma:
Fresh frozen plasma contains all coagulation factors at levels close to normal plasma levels. It is indicated to replace deficiencies of factors II, V, VII, IX, X, XI and antithrombin III. All coagulation factors, with the exception of factors V and VIII, are stable in whole blood. Factors V and VIII decrease to 15 and 50% respectively by 21 days of

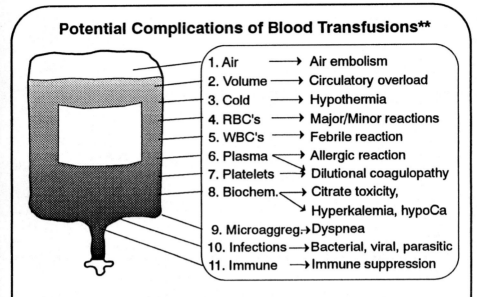

Potential Complications of Blood Transfusions**

1. Air	→→	Air embolism
2. Volume	→→	Circulatory overload
3. Cold	→→	Hypothermia
4. RBC's	→→	Major/Minor reactions
5. WBC's	→→	Febrile reaction
6. Plasma	⇄	Allergic reaction
7. Platelets	→↗	Dilutional coagulopathy
8. Biochem.	⤚	Citrate toxicity, Hyperkalemia, hypoCa
9. Microaggreg.	⇢	Dyspnea
10. Infections	→→	Bacterial, viral, parasitic
11. Immune	→→	Immune suppression

Figure 20.1: The components of whole blood all have potential side effects. By recalling the components of whole blood, one can readily recall their potential complications with their administration.

storage. However, only 20 percent of factor V, and 30% of factor VIII are needed for adequate hemostasis.

Packed RBCs, however, do not have adequate amounts of coagulation factors, and fresh frozen plasma is frequently useful in correcting deficiencies in factors V and VIII when transfusing multiple unitsts of packed RBCs. Fresh frozen plasma is also indicated in patients with liver disease who are bleeding and have multiple coagulation defects. Patients taking coumadin requiring emergency surgery may benefit from vitamin K_1 and FFP to correct their coagulation defect.

A dilutional coagulopathy may result when coagulation factor levels decrease. This occurs with a RBC transfusion equivalent to one blood volume ($\geq$ 10 units of PRBCs in adults). When the blood loss approaches one blood volume, in a patient with a previously normal coagulation status, fresh frozen plasma should be considered. Once fresh frozen plasma is required, one unit will be required for every two units of PRBCs.

Platelets:
Platelet transfusions are indicated after massive transfusion (> 1 blood volume transfused), associated with abnormal

bleeding and dilutional thrombocytopenia. Acute thrombocytopenia (platelet count 50,000 - 100,000 x 10^9/l) accompanied by microvascular bleeding is an indication for platelet transfusion. Platelets may be indicated prophylactically in the severely thrombocytopenic patient (e.g., thrombocytopenia secondary to chemotherapy). Patients with disorders resulting in platelet destruction or sequestration (e.g., hypersplenism) do not usually require platelet transfusions. The administration of one unit of platelets to an adult will raise the platelet count by approximately 5,000 - 10,000 x 10^9/l. Once platelet products are required, 1 - 2 units of platelets for every two units of PRBCs, are needed to maintain hemostasis.

Potential Complications of blood transfusions**:
The most common cause of an ABO incompatible transfusion results from a clerical error in patient and blood identification. Each unit must be checked prior to transfusion, preferably by two individuals. The patient's name and identification number must be identical to that on the unit of blood. The ABO and Rh type, blood product number, requisition number, expiry date, and any special precautions should also be checked.

Figure 20.1 lists the potential complications of blood transfusions. As ABO errors are the most common and serious errors made in the administration of blood products, it is prudent to know the patients ABO blood group and ensure this is correct before checking and administering blood. This simple

step becomes especially important when administering multiple units of blood. Figures 20.2 and 20.3 illustrate a simple method of checking the ABO compatability when type specific blood is not available and another ABO group must be used for blood product administration.

1. *Air:* During operative procedures when blood loss is brisk, the blood products may be pressurized to facilitate rapid administration. Whenever blood is administered under pressure, the risk of air embolism exists. Blood units that are now used to warm blood during rapid administration incorporate an air trap to minimize this risk.

2. *Volume:* Excessive administration of blood products may result in circulatory overload with pulmonary edema, and congestive heart failure.

3. *Cold:* The rapid administration of cold blood (massive transfusion) can result in a precipitous drop in the core body temperature. Ventricular dysrhythmias are more likely if the temperature drops below 30°C. The risk of ventricular fibrillation peaks at 28°C.

4. *RBCs:* Immediate hemolytic transfusion reactions are caused by the recipient's red cell antibodies (e.g., anti-A or anti-B) binding compliment and lysing the transfused RBCs. They are usually the result of an ABO incom-

patibility. The destruction occurs immediately, and as little as 20 ml may initiate a reaction. The reaction is characterized by severe signs and symptoms which may include: chills, fever, dyspnea, nausea, and chest or flank pain. Under anaesthesia, other signs such as hypotension, wheezing, hypoxemia, abnormal bleeding, and hemoglobinuria may be noted. Free hemoglobin is released from the lysed RBCs and is present in the urine and plasma (red urine and plasma). The most serious complications are acute renal failure (from the hemoglobin obstructing the tubules), and coagulopathy. Treatment includes:

A. Stop the blood immediately.
B. Notify the blood bank of the problem.
C. Send the remaining blood, as well as blood samples from the patient to the lab.
D. Send a urine sample for analysis (hemoglobinuria).
E. Administer oxygen.
F. Support the circulation (ephedrine, epinephrine, dopamine).
G. Promote a diuresis and renal excretion of hemoglobin by administering fluids, mannitol, furosemide, and/or dopamine. Consider alkalinizing the urine with intravenous sodium bicarbonate administration. Maintain a minimal urine output of 1 - 2 ml/kg/hr.
H. Monitor for disseminated intravascular coagulopathy (DIC). Follow the platelet count, fibrinogen level, INR, and PTT, and treat with plate-

lets, FFP, or cyroprecipitate as indicated.

RBCs: Delayed hemolytic transfusion reactions occur 2 - 21 days after the transfusion. Unlike the immediate ABO transfusion reaction, these reactions are often not preventable. They are usually due to trace antibodies formed after a previous transfusion or pregnancy. The concentration of these antibodies is so low they go undetected at the time of compatibility testing. The antibodies in the recipient's blood coat the transfused blood cells but do not result in immediate lysis. Later, the reticulo-endothelial system (RES) removes the cells from the circulation. The usual course is benign and often only detected because of the drop in hemoglobin and rise in bilirubin.

5. *WBCs:* White blood cells cause febrile reactions. These reactions may be accompanied by nausea, chills, headaches and myalgias. Less commonly, chest pain, hypotension, and vomiting may occur. Other causes of a fever during a transfusion includes major transfusion reactions (see above), reactions to platelets, and fever arising from bacterial contamination of the blood. Acetaminophen may be helpful in minor reactions. Occasionally, WBC filters, or WBC reduced blood products may be required if repeated febrile reactions occur.

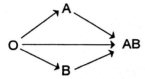

Packed RBC donation

Figure 20.2: Donors with ABO blood group O may donate packed RBC's to patients with blood group O, A, B, or AB, and are referred to as universal donors. Donors with the ABO blood group AB are only able to donate packed RBC's to AB recipients.

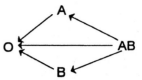

Plasma donation

Figure 20.3: Donors with ABO blood group O may receive plasma from donors with blood group O, A, B, or AB. However, patients with O blood, can only donate their plasma to patients with O type blood.

6. *Plasma:* A dilutional coagulopathy may result when coagulation factor levels decrease (see text above). Allergic reactions are due to foreign proteins in the blood. The most common manifestation of an allergic reaction is urticaria, which usually responds to antihistamines such as diphenhydramine (benadryl®). More severe reactions may result in an anaphylactic transfusion reaction with hypotension, and require the administration of corticosteroids, epinephrine, and fluids (see chapter 24: Unusual Anaesthetic Complications; Anaphylaxis). These patients may be found to be deficient in IgA and to have formed anti-IgA antibodies. Subsequent transfusions may require specific RBCs that are washed free of IgA.

7. *Platelets:* Dilutional thrombo-cytopenia with a platelet count of less than $100,000 \times 10^9/l$ occurs in over 90% of patients receiving 10 or more units of packed RBCs. This is the most common cause of a coagulopathy in a massively transfused patient.

8. *Biochemical abnormalities:* Rapid administration of packed RBCs (> 100 ml/minute) may result in citrate toxicity. Citrate is used as an anticoagulant in packed RBCs. Citrate binds calcium, producing hypocalcemia, decreased myocardial contractility, hypotension, and a widened QRS complex with a prolonged QT interval. Administration of calcium chloride 10 - 15 mg/kg, infused in slowly iv over 2 - 3 minutes, is indicated with documented hypocalcemia, or ECG changes accompanying hypotension.

Potassium concentrations of > 25 meq/l, with pH values of < 6.7 are normal values in stored packed RBCs. As the blood is transfused and the pH normalizes, the potassium rapidly shifts back into the RBC. Hence either hyperkalemia, or occasionally hypokalemia may be observed after a blood transfusion.

9. *Microaggregates:* Standard blood administration sets are equipped with 170 μm filters. They prevent small clots present in the donor units from being transfused and lodging in the pulmonary circulation. These filters should be used on RBC products, platelets, FFP, and cyroprecipitate. Microaggregates consist of platelets, WBCs, and fibrin which aggregate to form clumps in RBC products. Standard 170 μm blood filters, however, do not filter out microaggregates. Microaggregate filters (20 - 40 μm) are not recommended as their use has never been shown to reduce the incidence of respiratory distress syndrome following multiple transfusions.

10. *Infections:* The most common type of infection following a transfusion is viral. Screening tests for hepatitis C, HIV and HTLV-I depend upon detection of the antibody to the virus, which may not have formed, despite the presence of a viremia. Antibodies can take up to 1 year to reach detectable levels in the case of an HIV infection. Blood is also screened for hepatitis B and syphilis. Testing the blood for malaria, cytomegalovirus, Epstein-Bar virus (infectious mononucleosis) and many other potentially transmissible diseases, is not done unless specifically requested.

11. *Immune:* There is a non-specific suppression of the immune system that occurs after transfusing blood products. This property has been exploited to improve renal allograft survival. Adverse effects of the immuno-suppression may be associated with an increased risk of postoperative infections and recurrence of cancer.

References:

1. Transfusion Practices. Second edition 1992. American Society of Anesthesiologists Committee on Transfusion Medicine.

2. McIntyre, BG. Blood conservation and transfusion practices. Contemp Anaesth 1994; 4: 4-7.

3. Barash PG, Cullen BF, Stoelting RK. (ed.) In: Clinical anesthesia. Second edition. JB Lippincott Co. 1993.

4. Doyle DJ. Complications of blood transfusion. Contemp Anaesth 1994; 3:18 - 19.

5. Waxman K., et al. Hemodynamic and oxygen transport effects of pentastarch in burn resuscitation. Annals of surgery 1989; 29: 3.

Notes:

CHAPTER 21

Common Perioperative Problems

This chapter provides a general approach to common perioperative problems. Abnormalities in heart rate and blood pressure are common problems for which an organized approach in their initial management is essential. Tables 21.1 - 21.5 present the classification and differential diagnosis (Ddx.) of common hemodynamic problems. These tables may be used for reference, and are not to be memorized.

I	A common approach to emergency problems
II	Ddx. of Bradycardia
III	Ddx. of Tachycardia
IV	Ddx. of Hypertension
V	Ddx. of Hypotension and shock states.
VI	Nausea, emesis
VII	Confusion, agitation and delirium

I. A Common Approach to Emergency Problems.

Over the next few years of your medical training, you will undoubtedly be faced with emergency situations requiring your intervention. The following discussion of common problems aims to prepare you for this situation. This may occur on the ward, in the emergency department, or in a critical care setting such as the operating room.

For any resuscitation problem, a stepped 'ABC' (airway, breathing, circulation) approach is used.

1. **Evaluate and ensure the patient has an adequate and unobstructed airway.**

Maneuvers to resolve a partial or complete airway obstruction take precedence over any other interventions. The clinician must be able both to recognize an airway obstruction and utilize maneuvers to resolve it.

If the patient is not intubated:

Quickly assess whether the patient has an airway obstruction preventing them from breathing. In the unconscious patient maneuvers such as a chin lift, jaw thrust, removal of foreign bodies, and insertion of oral or nasal airways may be used to overcome an airway obstruction. Signs of an obstructed airway include lack of air movement despite respiratory efforts, noisy or stridorous respirations, intercostal indrawing, tracheal tugging, accessory muscle use, and lack of air entry on auscultation of the chest.

If the patient is intubated:

If the patient is intubated it is important quickly to ensure that the endotracheal tube is in fact in the trachea. Indirect confirmation includes listening for equal air entry to both lung fields and observing chest excursion during positive pressure ventilation. You should be able to pass a suction catheter through the tracheal tube without meeting any obstruction. Finally, epigastric auscultation should be negative for air entry to the stomach during positive pressure ventilation. A portable chest X-ray can be used to confirm that the tip of the tube is in the mid-trachea.

Direct confirmation that the tracheal tube is in the trachea can be immediately obtained by visualizing the tube passing through the glottis during direct laryngoscopy. When doubt exists concerning the positioning of the tracheal tube or its patency, a fiberoptic bronchoscope can be passed through the tube into the trachea. Observing carbon dioxide returning with each exhaled breath (end-tidal CO_2 monitoring) provides immediate confirmation of tracheal intubation.

2. Evaluate and ensure that the patient is receiving adequate oxygen.

In any emergency situation, it is always wise to apply oxygen. The Ambu bag and mask provide a rapid method of providing 100% oxygen. It allows the patient to breathe 100% oxygen with the option of assisting their spontaneous efforts. Manual ventilation can be administered with this device when the patient is not breathing (see figure 23.4).

Examine the patient. Is there evidence of cyanosis? Quickly scan any monitors attached to the patient. Ask for assistance in applying monitors such as a blood pressure cuff, ECG monitor, and pulse oximeter. Ensure that oxygen is being delivered from the source to the patient.

3. Evaluate and ensure the patients ventilation is adequate.

There are many conditions that can result in respiratory insufficiency. Ventilation must be provided when a patient is not breathing. Auscultation, palpation, and percussion of the chest, in combination with the vital signs and pulse oximetry, are used in the immediate evaluation of the patient. Arterial blood gas analysis, chest X-ray, and pulmonary function tests may also be required to formulate a working diagnosis of the etiology of the respiratory insufficiency.

4. Assess the heart rate and rhythm.

Quickly confirm or rule out an arrest situation.
*Severe bradycardia must be assumed to be secondary to hypoxemia until proven otherwise***.

5. Assess the blood pressure and perfusion.

Hypotension may result in decreased organ perfusion. Clinical findings that are associated with decreased organ perfusion include:

CNS: anxiety
confusion
unconsciousness
CVS: dysrhythmias or ECG
evidence of ischemia
Renal: decreased urine output.

The blood pressure should be confirmed by a manual cuff if there is any question concerning its validity. Arterial lines, automated blood pressure cuffs, and human error can all be responsible for factitious blood pressures.

6. Assess the patients volume status.

Important changes in a patient's blood volume status may be clinically subtle. Significant alterations in vital signs and mental status may result. Assess the jugular venous pressure and the patients recent urine output. In the operating room, it would be appropriate to review the patient's duration of fasting, examine the surgical wound, sponges, suction apparatus, and nasogastric drainage. An overall assessment of the blood losses, and third space losses as well as the adequacy of fluid replacement should be made (see chapter 20: Intravenous and Blood Component Therapy).

7. Check the patients temperature.

Alterations in temperature associated with anaesthesia and surgery may result in important cardiorespiratory abnormalities. Both hypothermia and hyperthermia may occur. Hypothermia is frequently the result of intraoperative

temperature losses. Temperature losses result from evaporative, conductive, radiant and convective loss of body heat. Patients undergoing surgery are exposed to a cold operating room with cold instruments, intravenous fluids and an open wound through which heat loss occurs. The resulting hypothermia may result in postoperative shivering, with a rise in heart rate, blood pressure and 5 to 6-fold increase in oxygen consumption. Increases in temperature perioperatively may result from drugs such as atropine, or from the administration of blood products. Other causes of an increased temperature include fever, sepsis, active intraoperative warming efforts, and underlying disease states such as thyrotoxicosis or malignant hyperthermia.

8. Scan for obvious causes of the abnormality.

Correct any obvious underlying abnormality. Hypotension and tachycardia with inadequate fluid replacement, and hypertension and tachycardia with inadequate analgesia are common examples. Scan any monitors that are attached to the patient, and consider establishing a large bore intravenous.

9. Establish additional monitors where appropriate.

Examples of additional monitors that may be appropriate include an ECG monitor, blood pressure cuff, pulse oximeter, and temperature probe. Invasive monitors may include a foley catheter, arterial line, central venous pressure line or pulmonary artery catheter.

10. Investigate.

Common investigations that may aid in confirming the diagnosis include a CBC, INR, PTT, ABG, CXR, ECG, glucose, electrolytes, and creatinine.

11. Formulate a plan, and recruit additional help if necessary.

In an emergency situation, you may not have the luxury of having an extensive history before you are required to act. Nevertheless, you can proceed with assessing the status of the patient's airway, oxygenation, ventilation, heart rate, rhythm, and blood pressure. Once the patient is hemodynamically stable and receiving adequate oxygen and ventilation, review the patient's history, recent lab data, perioperative course (in the case of recent surgery), and formulate a provisional diagnosis so that you may initiate treatment. Remember to recruit help in any emergency.

II - IV: Tables 21.1 to 21.3 list the causes of alterations in heart rate and increases in blood pressure perioperatively.

V: Hypotension

The purpose of the cardiopulmonary circulation is to deliver oxygen and nutrients to body tissues. When tissue needs are not met, a state of shock is said to exist. The blood pressure is used as a gross indirect measurement of organ perfusion and assessment of the adequacy of the circulation. It represents a complex interaction between cardiac output, blood volume and systemic vascular resistance (SVR). The cardiac output is determined by the heart rate, preload, contractility and afterload (SVR).

In a normal adult, hypotension is generally defined as a systolic blood pressure of less than 90 mm Hg, or a mean arterial pressure of less than 60 mm Hg. The most common cause of a hypotensive state is a decrease in intravascular volume. This may result from an acute hemorrhage or from a loss of fluids and electrolytes (see table 20.3: Common conditions associated with fluid deficits). Acute hypovolemia reduces the venous return to the heart (preload) resulting in a decrease in cardiac output and systemic blood pressure. Carotid and aortic baroreceptors sense the decrease in arterial pressure, and initiate a series of events resulting in an increase in sympathetic output from the central nervous system and adrenal gland. The resulting release of norepinephrine and epinephrine increase the heart rate, contractility and SVR in an effort to redirect and maintain blood flow to vital organs.

Hypovolemic shock is the most common type of shock. A low central venous pressure and low pulmonary capillary wedge pressure (PCWP) is diagnostic of hypovolemia. Other forms of circulatory shock include distributive shock, obstructive shock and cardiogenic shock. Table 21.4 characterizes the hemodynamic features of the different forms of shock.

Table 21.1: Differential Diagnosis of a Decreased Heart Rate		
RESP	Hypoxemia Hypercarbia	Acidosis
CVS	**Congenital Heart Block** **Increased Parasympathetic tone:** - Vagal reflexes (see CNS) - Drugs - Paediatric patients	**Decreased Sympathetic Tone:** - Beta Blockers - High spinal or epidural anaesthesia (> T1 - T4) - Neurogenic shock
	Decreased Conduction: - Sinus bradycardia - Junctional bradycardia - Idioventricular escape rhythm - Sick Sinus Syndrome	- Atrial Fibrillation with a slow ventricular response - Type II Second degree AV block - Complete Heart Block - Ventricular Asystole
CNS	**Baroreceptor reflex** secondary to increased blood pressure or increased ICP	
	Vagal Reflexes: - Vasovagal reflex - oculocardiac reflex - carotid sinus reflex - airway manipulation (especially important in paediatric patients)	**Drugs:** - Anaesthetic overdose - Succinylcholine - Opioids - Edrophonium, neostigmine - Halothane - Digoxin - Beta blockers
Other	Hypothermia Hypothyroidism	Athlete
℞	**Treatment options** might include: - oxygen - fluids - Trendelenburg position - remove offending cause - treat underlying drug toxicity (eg. Digibind for digoxin toxicity)	- atropine - ephedrine - isuprel - epinephrine - transcutaneous or transvenous pacemaker - cardiopulmonary resuscitation

Distributive shock is characterized by systemic vasodilation, relative hypovolemia and an increase in cardiac output. The most common form of distributive shock is septic shock. Arteriovenous shunting at the tissue level results in an accumulation of lactic acid and tissue anoxia. Table 21.4 lists

Table 21.2:	Differential Diagnosis of an Increased Heart Rate	
RESP	Hypoxia Hypercarbia Acidosis	
CVS	**Sinus Tachycardia:** A reflex sinus tachycardia may occur in shock states (see Table 21.5: Classification of Shock States). Sinus tachycardia may arise due to decreases in preload, afterload or contractility. Increased sympathetic stimulation arising from anxiety, pain, drugs and surgical stress is a common cause of sinus tachycardia. **Other rhythms:** - paroxysmal atrial tachycardia (PAT) - accelerated junctional rhythm - multifocal atrial tachycardia (eg. COPD patient) - atrial flutter with or without heart block - atrial fibrillation - pre-excitation syndromes with accessory pathways - ventricular tachycardia	
CNS	Awareness under anaesthesia Anxiety Pain	
GU	Full bladder	
HEME	Anemia Transfusion reaction	
ENDO	**Hypermetabolic states:** - fever - sepsis - pheochromocytoma - thyrotoxicosis - malignant hyperthermia - malignant neuroleptic syndrome	**Other:** - Addisonian crisis - porphyria - hypoglycemia - hypercalcemia
IMMUNE	Anaphylaxis	
DRUGS	Atropine Cocaine (used for local anaesthesia) Dopamine Epinephrine	Ephedrine Isoflurane Isoproterenol Pancuronium
Treatment is directed at the underlying cause of the increased heart rate.		

examples of the four classes of shock.

Cardiogenic shock results when the heart fails to perform its pumping function. This occurs as a result of a myocardial, valvular, or electrical

Table 21.3:	Differential Diagnosis of an Increased Blood Pressure Perioperatively		
RESP	Hypoxia Hypercarbia		
CVS	Essential hypertension Coarctation Post-carotid endarterectomy (acute denervation of carotid baroreceptors)		
CNS	Pain Shivering Hypothermia Anxiety	Full bladder Light Anaesthetic level Emergence delirium Increased ICP	Autonomic mass reflex (quadraparetic or paraplegic patients)
GU	Renal artery stenosis Parenchymal Disease Pregnancy induced hypertension Toxemia		
ENDO	Hyperthyroidism Cushings disease or syndrome Pheochromocytoma Conn's syndrome (hyperaldosteronism)	Carcinoid Hyperparathyroidism - hypercalcemia	
MSK	Malignant hyperthermia Malignant neuroleptic syndrome		
DRUGS	Ephedrine Epinephrine Cocaine Phenylephrine Ketamine Acute narcotic reversal with naloxone Drug interactions: - Monoamine oxidase inhibitors (MAOI's) with meperidine - MAOI's with indirect acting vasopressors (eg. ephedrine)	Rebound from stopping antihypertensive drugs: - clonidine - beta blockers	
Treatment is directed at the underlying cause of the increased blood pressure.			

problem. A myocardial infarction is the most common cause of cardiogenic shock. Characteristic findings include an increase in CVP, PCWP, and SVR, with a cardiac index of less than 1.8 L/min/m^2 and a systolic BP less than 80 mm Hg (see table 10.1 and 10.2 for derivations and normal values).

Table 21.4:			Hemodynamic Parameters		
Shock State	BP	CVP	PCWP	CO	SVR
Hypovolemic	↓	↓	↓	↓	↑
Cardiogenic - (LV dysfunction) - (RV Infarction)	↓ ↓	↑ ↑	↑↑ (> 20 mm Hg) ↓	↓ ↓	↑↑ ↑↑
Distributive	↓	↓	↓	↑	↓↓
Obstructive	↓	↑	↑ or ↓	↓	↑

Obstructive shock occurs when there is an obstruction preventing cardiac filling or emptying. Two immediately treatable causes of obstructive shock include a tension pneumothorax and cardiac tamponade.

Hemorrhagic Shock Classification:
The normal response to increasing hemorrhage produces characteristic physiological signs. These signs have been used to classify hemorrhagic shock according to the quantity of blood loss. Table 21.6 defines 4 classes of hemorrhagic shock based on the patient's vital signs, and predicts the percent blood loss and appropriate initial therapy.

Class I hemorrhage:
Defined as the loss of as much as 15% of blood volume. It is associated with minimal physiologic changes.

Class II hemorrhage:
Defined as a 15 - 30% loss of blood volume. Class II hemorrhage is associated with modest elevations in heart rate and decreases in pulse pressure as diastolic pressures rise with smaller stroke volumes. Systolic pressures tend to be maintained, but digital capillary refill is slightly retarded. Urinary output is only mildly depressed. Postural hypotension may be associated with class II hemorrhage, as may subtle central nervous system changes such as fright and hostility.

Class III hemorrhage:
Defined as a 30 - 40% loss of blood volume. Patients with class III hemorrhage present with tachycardia, systolic and diastolic hypotension, delayed capillary refill (>2 seconds), reduced urinary output, and an apprehensive, slightly clouded sensorium.

Class IV hemorrhage:
Defined as a blood loss of 40% or more of the blood volume. The patient manifests signs of frank shock with cool, diaphoretic, ashen skin, tachycardia, hypotension or unobtainable blood pressure, anuria, and a reduced level of consciousness.

Patients with class III and IV hemorrhages will require immediate intravenous fluid administration to survive. Patients with class IV hemorrhage

Table 21.5:	Classification and Etiology of Shock States
Hypovolemic Shock	
- most common cause of shock	- occult blood or fluid losses
Cardiogenic Shock	
Myocardial: - relative drug overdose (anaesthetic drugs) - other drug effects (β-blocker, Ca^{2+} channel blocker) - ischemia - infarction - rupture (papillary muscle, ventricular septum, chordae tendonae)	Myocardial (continued): - arrhythmias - cardiomyopathy (congestive, hypertrophic, restrictive, or obliterative) Valvular Disease: (esp. NB when stress is superimposed) Aortic regurgitation Mitral regurgitation
Distributive Shock	
Anaphylaxis, Anaphylactoid reaction Sepsis Drugs (Vasodilators) Neurogenic shock High regional sympathectomy (eg. high spinal anaesthesia)	Addisonian crisis Transfusion reaction Severe liver disease A - V fistulas Thyrotoxicosis Hypothyroidism
Obstructive Shock	
Tension pneumothorax Pericardial tamponade Pulmonary embolism (blood clot, fat, air, tumor, etc) Supine hypotension during pregnancy (aortocaval compression gravid uterus) IVC, or heart compression by surgical instruments	Aortic dissection Aortic cross-clamping Atrial myxoma IHSS Valvular heart disease with stress (eg. Aortic or mitral stenosis with pregnancy or trauma).

will require blood transfusion to survive, but class III hemorrhage patients may tolerate post-resuscitation anemia if fluid resuscitation is accompanied with immediate control of the hemorrhage.

Hematocrits as low as 20 to 25% may be well tolerated if total blood volume is adequate. The use of clinical signs to estimate traumatic blood loss is very important because soft tissues and body

Table 21.6:		Classification of Hemorrhagic Shock	
Hemorrhage	**% Blood Volume loss**	**Physiological changes.**	**Treatment**
Class I	≤ 15	HR < 100/min. SBP normal PP:normal or increased CR: normal RR: 14 - 20/min. CNS: Anxious	Rapidly infuse 1 - 2 liters of balanced salt solution (BSS), then maintenance fluids.
Class II	15 - 30	HR > 100/min. SBP normal DBP increased Postural hypotension PP: decreased CR: delayed RR: 20 - 30/min. CNS: more anxious	Rapidly infuse 2 liters of BSS, re-evaluate continued needs
Class III	30 - 40	HR > 120/min. SBP decreased PP: decreased CR: delayed or absent RR: 30 - 40/min. CNS: Confused	Rapidly infuse 2 liters of BSS; re-evaluate; replace blood losses with 1:3 BSS or 1:1 with blood (PRBC's, colloid, other blood products). Maintain urine output > 0.5 ml/kg/hr.
Class IV	≥ 40	HR > 140/min. SBP decreased PP: decreased CR: absent RR > 35/min. CNS: Lethargic	

HR = heart rate (bpm); SBP = systolic blood pressure; DBP = diastolic blood pressure; PP = pulse pressure; CR = capillary refill; RR = respiratory rate; CNS = central nervous system

cavities frequently conceal large quantities of blood with minimal external body changes.

VI: Nausea and vomiting.

Nausea and vomiting, have a profound effect on the patients perception of their perioperative care. It has been shown to significantly increase the time the patient spends in the post anaesthetic care unit (PACU), and places the patient who is recovering from anaesthesia at risk of gastric aspiration.

Preoperative patient risk factors include:

1. Previous history of anaesthetic associated nausea and vomiting (review old chart if possible).
2. Young age.
3.. Female gender. (The probability of postoperative nausea and vomiting has been linked to a woman's menstrual cycle.)
4. Operative procedure. (Increased incidence with eye, middle ear, and female pelvic surgery).
5. Obesity.

Many anaesthetic agents have been associated with nausea and vomiting. The mechanisms are multiple and complex. Opioids are perhaps the most potent emetics. They have been shown to directly stimulate the chemoreceptor trigger zone of the fourth ventricle, stimulate the vestibular apparatus, delay gastric emptying, and increase gastric secretions.

Nitrous oxide may have a direct action on the chemoreceptor trigger zone, as well as acting on the middle ear, and cause both gastric and bowel distension. Other common agents associated with perioperative nausea include sodium thiopental, inhalational agents, and cholinesterase inhibitors.

Nausea and vomiting perioperatively must be assumed to be secondary to bradycardia and hypotension until proven otherwise**.

When assessing a patient with perioperative nausea and vomiting, quickly evaluate the patients vital signs. Vagal reflexes, with a decrease in blood pressure and heart rate, may present as nausea and vomiting.

A differential diagnosis for nausea and vomiting includes:
Hypotension
Bradycardia
Drug induced nausea
  - opioids
  - anaesthetic agents
Surgical manipulation
Pain
  - surgical
  - biliary or renal colic
  - migraine
Drug toxicity:
  - digoxin
  - theophylline
  - ASA
  - alcohol
Hyponatremia
  - postoperative TURP patients
Hypercalcemia
  - cancer patients
Diabetic ketoacidosis
Pregnancy
Coexisting gastroenteritis
Acute hepatitis
Other:
  - renal failure
  - hepatic failure
  - adrenal failure
  - hypothyroidism
  - raised ICP

There is no one treatment for this problem. Frequently a number of factors contribute to the patient's nausea. Switching the opioid used for postoperative analgesia, or adding a non steroidal anti-inflammatory agent may resolve the problem.

Common agents used to treat perioperative nausea and vomiting include:

Droperidol†
  0.25 - 0.5 mg iv prn
Dimenhydrinate (Gravol®)
  10 - 50 mg iv/im/po
  (maximum 50 mg q 3 - 4 hours).
Metochlorpropamide†
  10 - 20 mg iv every 6 hours prn.
  (contraindicated in bowel obstruction)
Prochlorperazine (Stemetil®)†
  10 mg im every 6 hours prn.

† Dopamine receptor antagonists. The potential for extrapyramidal reactions increases as dosage and number of agents used increase. Dysphoric reactions and disturbed sleep patterns have been reported with moderate doses of droperidol (2.5 mg iv).

Less common agents used include:
Propofol 10 mg iv.
One mg/kg/hr infusions have been used successfully to prevent nausea and vomiting in patients receiving chemotherapy, who have a past history of nausea and vomiting.

Ondansetron is a new selective serotonin antagonist. It is more commonly used to treat radiation or chemotherapy-related nausea and vomiting. An oral dose of 8 mg may be administered one hour prior to anaesthesia in patients with a history of resistant nausea and vomiting associated with anaesthesia. This is followed by 2 additional doses of 8 mg each at 8 hour intervals. Alternatively, established nausea and vomiting may respond to a single injection of 4 mg intravenously.

A combination of antiemetic drugs may be more effective in preventing postoperative nausea and vomitting. The combination of ondansetron and dexamethasone has been shown to be effective in reducing the incidence of nausea and vomitting in cisplatin chemotherapy. Ondasetron (4mg) and dexamethasone (8 mg) has recently shown promising results in preventing nausea and vomitting postoperatively[4].

VII: Postoperative Agitation and delirium.

The agitated, delirious, or aggressive patient is rarely seen in the PACU today. This is due perhaps to a combination of our improved understanding of pain management, the availability of shorter-acting anaesthetic agents, and improvements in our monitoring equipment (oximetry, peripheral nerve stimulator, and end-tidal carbon dioxide monitoring).

An initial ABC approach is used, with the use of physical restraints if needed to protect both the patient and the medical team. The physical restraints are removed as soon as the offending cause is removed or chemical restraints substituted.

Upper airway obstruction, residual paralysis, hypercarbia, and hypoxemia are all potent stimulants which can produce an agitated state**.

A gross neurological examination should be performed quickly (e.g., pupillary assessment, movement of arms and legs, Glasgow coma scale (GCS) score), while communicating reassuringly with the patient.

Elderly patients are particularly prone to postoperative confusion and agitation. Common causes of agitation include pain and bladder or bowel distension. Patients recovering from anaesthesia may appear able to communicate verbally, but unable to recognize that the cause of their distress is pain or a full bladder.

Less common causes of an agitated postoperative state include:
Drug effect
  - ketamine
  - anticholinergics:
    - atropine
    - scopolamine
    - tricyclic antidepressants
TURP syndrome
  - hyponatremia
  - glycine toxicity
Hypercalcemia
  - cancer patients
Hypoglycemia
Acute Stroke
Raised ICP
Anxiety
Fear
Separation from caregivers
Acute drug withdrawal
Acute drug intoxication

Following clinical evaluation, appropriate investigations may include a measurement of the patient's glucose, electrolytes, calcium, arterial blood gas, and tests of neuromuscular strength.

If a thorough search fails to identify any of the above causes of postoperative agitation, small doses of a benzodiazepine such as midazolam (0.5 - 1.0 mg iv), or an antipsychotic such as haldol (2.5 - 5.0 mg iv/im) may be warranted.

Consider small doses of:
Naloxone (0.04 - 0.08 mg increments)
Flumazenil (0.2 - 0.6 mg iv), or
Physostigmine (0.5 - 2 mg iv)
respectively, if excessive sedation is felt to be secondary to opioids, benzodiazepines, or anticholinergic agents.

References:

1. Review Article: Anaesthesia and emesis. I, II. Palazzo MGA, Strunin L. Can Anaesth. Soc. J. 1984; 31: 178-87, 407-15.

2. Review Article: Postoperative nausea and vomiting: Its etiology, treatment and prevention. Watcha MF, White PF. Anesthesiology 1992; 77: 162-84.

3. Larijani GE, GratzI, Afsar M, Minassian S. Anesth Analg 1991; 73; 246-9.

4. Rajeeva V, Bhardwaj N, Batra YK, Dhaliwal LK. Can J Anesth 1999; 46: 40 - 44.

Notes:

CHAPTER 22

Managing the Circulation

Hemodynamic abnormalities of the circulation may necessitate interventions to maintain normal oxygen transport and organ perfusion. This may occur in the perioperative period as a result of pain, anxiety, hypoxia, hypercarbia, and abnormalities of temperature or intravascular volume (see chapter 21). Correcting these abnormalities should precede the administration of any vasoactive agents.

Pharmacologic manipulation of both the parasympathetic and sympathetic nervous systems may be required to correct hypotensive, ischemic or hypertensive emergencies. Table 22.1 lists the different classes of medications that may be used to restore circulatory homeostasis.

Central to our understanding of the circulation and oxygen transport is the concept of cardiac output. The *cardiac output (CO)* is defined as the amount of blood pumped to the peripheral circulation per minute. It is expressed as the product of the heart rate multiplied by the stroke volume.

$$CO = HR \; x \; SV$$

A normal CO value for an adult is 2.5 to 3.5 L/min/m², or 4.5 to 6.0 L/min in a 70 kg adult. The CO can increase by a factor of 10 during extreme exercise in normal adults. The three determinants of the stroke volume are the *preload, afterload, and contractility.*

The *preload* is defined as the end-diastolic stretch of the left ventricle. As preload increases so does the left ventricular work, cardiac output, blood pressure, and stroke volume (recall the Frank-Starling curves). Excessive increases in end-diastole stretch results in a decline in cardiac performance when the left ventricle becomes overdistended. The left ventricular end-diastolic volume (LVEDV) is our best measurement of preload. Since the LVEDV is difficult to measure clinically, the filling pressures of the left ventricle at end-diastole (LVEDP) may be estimated by the measuring the pulmonary capillary wedge pressure (PCWP) with a pulmonary artery catheter. Generally, an increase in the LVEDP corresponds with an increase in LVEDV. In patients with normal a right and left ventricle, mitral valve, pulmonary vasculature, and airway pressures, the assessment of the central venous pressure (CVP) may be used to estimate the LVEDV and preload.

Afterload is defined as the myocardial wall stress of the left ventricle during ejection. It is a measure of the work the left ventricle performs with each contraction. In the absence of aortic stenosis, afterload depends on the elasticity of the large arteries and on the systemic vascular resistance (SVR). The SVR can be estimated using a calculation incorporating the mean arterial blood pressure, cardiac output, and CVP (see table 10.1 and 10.2).

Contractility is the myocardium's intrinsic ability to perform work at any given level of end-diastolic fiber length (preload). It is primarily determined by the availability of intracellular calcium. All agents that increase myocardial contractility produce an increase in intracellular calcium. Contractility increases with sympathetic stimulation and inotropic drugs, such as digoxin. Hypoxia, acidosis, beta blockers, calcium channel blockers, and myocardial ischemia or infarction are common conditions that depress contractility. Increases in preload, heart rate, contractility or decreases in afterload, all promote forward flow and an increase in cardiac output.

Vasoactive drugs may be classified as acting by either a catecholamine or a non-catecholamine mechanism. Drugs acting through a catecholamine mechanism may have either agonist or antagonist receptor activity. Most catecholamine vasoactive drugs have a combination of alpha and beta adrenergic receptor activity (see tables 22.3 - 22.5). When choosing to use a vasoactive medication, one ought to consider the risks of using the drug, the hemodynamic goals one seeks, and the pharmacologic properties of the drug.

Patients presenting to, or leaving the operating room with vasoactive medications infusing, must be considered to be seriously ill. All vasoactive agents have serious potential side effects that must be considered whenever they are used. Indiscriminate infusions of vasopressors may produce the desired increase in blood pressure, but may also severely restrict blood flow to vital organs such as the bowel, liver and kidney. Marked increases in peripheral vascular resistance produced by vasopressors may precipitate cardiac failure.

The principle goal of circulatory support is to optimize tissue perfusion with oxygenated blood. To achieve this, one must assess and optimize the preload, afterload, heart rate, contractility, oxygen transport and organ perfusion (see table below).

Optimize	Assessed by:
Preload	PCWP: 10 - 15 mmHg CVP: 8 - 12 mmHg
Afterload	SVR = 900 - 1500 dynes·sec·cm^{-5}
Contractility	CI > 2.5 L/min/m^2
Heart Rate	60 - 90 bpm
Oxygen Transport	Arterial blood gas Mixed venous oxygen saturation (MvO$_2$) Hemoglobin
Organ Perfusion	MvO$_2$ saturation Serum lactate ABG Urine output CNS sensorium

Table 22.1: Cardiorespiratory effects of receptor stimulation.

Receptors	Agonist	Antagonist
Adrenergic: Alpha-1	Vasoconstriction of the skin, gut, kidney, liver, and heart (e.g., phenylephrine).	Peripheral vasodilation, reflex tachycardia, hypotension (e.g., prazosin)
Alpha-2	Reduces sympathetic outflow from the CNS inhibiting norepinephrine release (e.g., clonidine, dexametomidine).	CNS stimulation, increased sympathetic outflow. Increased HR, contractility, and cardiac output.
Beta-1	Increased heart rate, myocardial conduction, and contractility (e.g., isoproterenol)	Decreased HR, contractility, and conduction, (e.g., esmolol).
Beta-2	Bronchodilation, peripheral vascular smooth muscle relaxation, (e.g., salbutamol).	Bronchospasm, peripheral vasoconstricton.
Dopamine-1	Peripheral vasodilation of the renal and splanchnic vasculature, (e.g., dopamine).	
Cholinergic (Muscarinic)	Decreases heart rate, conduction, and cardiac output. Increases bronchial secretions, (e.g., edrophonium).	Anticholinergics increase heart rate, conduction, and contractility. They also decrease bronchial secretions, (e.g., atropine).
Calcium channel	Increases contractility, vasoconstriction (e.g., calcium).	Decreases contractility, increases vasodilation, (e.g., nifedipine).
Other	Phosphodiesterase inhibitors: Produce a concentration dependant increase in contractility with arterial and venous dilation (e.g., amrinone). Cardiac glycosides: (e.g., digoxin)	

Table 22.2: Manipulating the determinants of cardiac output to correct hemodynamic disturbances in the circulation. Tables 21.1 - 21.6 are presented for reference only.

Determinants of Cardiac Output	Hemodynamic Disturbance (accompanied by lists of vasoactive agents and interventions used to treat the disturbance)	
Preload	**Increased Preload** Venous vasodilators - nitroglycerine - nitroprusside Diuretics - furosemide Phlebotomy	**Decreased Preload** Crystalloid, colloid infusion (see chapter 20)
Heart Rate	**Increased Heart Rate** Beta blockers - propranolol - metoprolol - esmolol Calcium channel blockers - verapamil	**Decreased Heart Rate** Anticholinergics - atropine Beta Agonists - isoproterenol - ephedrine Pacemaker
Contractility	**Increased contractility** General anaesthetics - halothane Beta blockers Calcium channel blockers	**Decreased Contractility** Digoxin Norepinephrine Amrinone Epinephrine Dopamine Surgery Ephedrine Intra-aortic Dobutamine balloon pump
Afterload	**Increased afterload** Arterial vasodilators - sodium nitroprusside - hydralazine Labetalol Amrinone ACE inhibitors - captopril - enalapril - lisinopril Dobutamine	**Decreased afterload** Alpha agonists - phenylephrine - norepinephrine Crystalloid or colloid fluid therapy

In October 1992, the National Conference on Cardiopulmonary Resuscitation (CPR) published the current recommendations for adult cardiac life support (ACLS). A summary of the algorithms are presented (for reference) in figures 22.1 to 22.5.

The Guidelines for Cardiopulmonary Resuscitation published in JAMA in 1992 classified therapeutic interventions as:

Class I: Recommendation is *definitely helpful*.

Class IIa: Recommendation acceptable, and *probably helpful*.

Class IIb: Recommendation acceptable and *possibly helpful*.

Class III: Recommendation is not indicated, and may be *harmful*.

The properties of vasoactive medications used in manipulating circulatory abnormalities are presented (for reference) in tables 22.3 to 22.7.

References:

1. Hug CC, Kaplan JA: Pharmacology - cardiac drugs, Cardiac Anesthesia, Edited by Kaplan JA.   Grune and Straton, 1979, pp 39 - 69.

2. Thys DM, Kaplan JA.   Cardiovascular physiology, Anesthesia, third ed. Edited by Miller RD.   Churchill Livingstone 1990, pp 551 - 583.

3. Merin RG.   Autonomic nervous system pharmacology,   Anesthesia third ed.   Edited by Miller RD. Churchill Livingstone 1990, pp 471 - 504.

4. American heart association: Textbook of advanced cardiac life support. 1992.

5. Emergency Cardiac Care Committee and Subcommittees, American Heart Association.   Guidelines for cardiopulmonary resuscitation and emergency cardiac care, III: Adult Advanced Cardiac Life Support. JAMA 1992; 268: 2199-241.

Footnotes for figure 22.1, page 213:

a. Unstable condition must be related to the tachycardia. Signs and symptoms may include chest pain, shortness of breath, decreased level of consciousness, low blood pressure (BP), shock, pulmonary congestion, congestive heart failure, acute myocardial infarction.

b. Carotid sinus pressure is contraindicated in patients with carotid bruits; avoid ice water immersion in patients with ischemic heart disease.

c. If the wide-complex tachycardia is known with certainty to be PSVT and BP is normal/elevated, sequence can include verapamil.

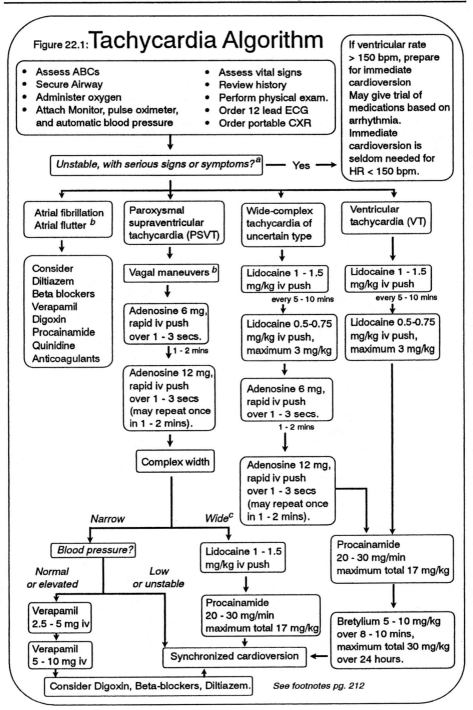

Figure 22.1: Tachycardia Algorithm

- Assess ABCs
- Secure Airway
- Administer oxygen
- Attach Monitor, pulse oximeter, and automatic blood pressure

- Assess vital signs
- Review history
- Perform physical exam.
- Order 12 lead ECG
- Order portable CXR

If ventricular rate > 150 bpm, prepare for immediate cardioversion. May give trial of medications based on arrhythmia. Immediate cardioversion is seldom needed for HR < 150 bpm.

Unstable, with serious signs or symptoms?[a] — Yes →

Atrial fibrillation Atrial flutter [b]

Consider
Diltiazem
Beta blockers
Verapamil
Digoxin
Procainamide
Quinidine
Anticoagulants

Paroxysmal supraventricular tachycardia (PSVT)

Vagal maneuvers [b]

Adenosine 6 mg, rapid iv push over 1 - 3 secs.
↓ 1 - 2 mins

Adenosine 12 mg, rapid iv push over 1 - 3 secs (may repeat once in 1 - 2 mins).

Complex width

Wide-complex tachycardia of uncertain type

Lidocaine 1 - 1.5 mg/kg iv push
every 5 - 10 mins

Lidocaine 0.5-0.75 mg/kg iv push, maximum 3 mg/kg

Adenosine 6 mg, rapid iv push over 1 - 3 secs.
1 - 2 mins

Adenosine 12 mg, rapid iv push over 1 - 3 secs (may repeat once in 1 - 2 mins).

Ventricular tachycardia (VT)

Lidocaine 1 - 1.5 mg/kg iv push
every 5 - 10 mins

Lidocaine 0.5-0.75 mg/kg iv push, maximum 3 mg/kg

Procainamide 20 - 30 mg/min maximum total 17 mg/kg

Narrow

Blood pressure?

Normal or elevated   *Low or unstable*

Wide[c]

Lidocaine 1 - 1.5 mg/kg iv push

Procainamide 20 - 30 mg/min maximum total 17 mg/kg

Verapamil 2.5 - 5 mg iv

Verapamil 5 - 10 mg iv

Bretylium 5 - 10 mg/kg over 8 - 10 mins, maximum total 30 mg/kg over 24 hours.

Synchronized cardioversion

Consider Digoxin, Beta-blockers, Diltiazem.   *See footnotes pg. 212*

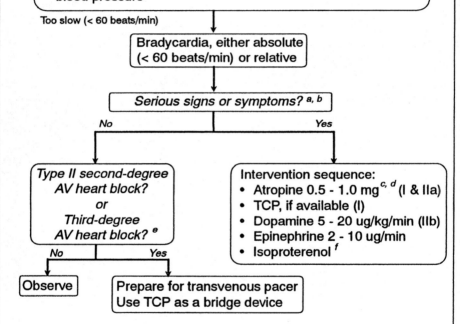

Figure 22.2: # Bradycardia algorithm
(Patient is not in cardiac arrest)

- Assess ABCs
- Secure airway
- Administer oxygen
- Start iv
- Attach monitor, pulse oximeter, and automatic blood pressure

- Assess vital signs
- Review history
- Perform physical examination
- Order 12 lead ECG
- Order portable CXR

Too slow (< 60 beats/min)

Bradycardia, either absolute (< 60 beats/min) or relative

Serious signs or symptoms? [a, b]

No   Yes

Type II second-degree AV heart block?
or
Third-degree AV heart block? [e]

No   Yes

Observe

Prepare for transvenous pacer
Use TCP as a bridge device

Intervention sequence:
- Atropine 0.5 - 1.0 mg [c, d] (I & IIa)
- TCP, if available (I)
- Dopamine 5 - 20 ug/kg/min (IIb)
- Epinephrine 2 - 10 ug/min
- Isoproterenol [f]

Footnotes for bradycardia algorithm:
a. *Serious signs or symptoms must be related to the slow rate. Clinical manifestations include chest pain, shortness of breath, decreased level of consciousness, low BP, shock, pulmonary congestion, CHF, acute myocardial infarction.*
b. *Do not delay TCP while awaiting iv access or for atropine to take effect if patient is symptomatic.*
c. *Denervated transplanted hearts will not respond to atropine. Go at once to pacing, catecholamine infusion, or both.*
d. *Atropine should be given in repeat doses in 3 - 5 min intervals up to 0.04 mg/kg. Consider shorter dosing intervals in severe conditions.*
e. *Never treat third-degree heart block plus ventricular escape beats with lidocaine.*
f. *Isoproterenol should be used, if at all, with extreme caution. At low doses it is Class IIb (possibly helpful); at higher doses it is Class III (harmful).*
g. *Verify patient tolerance and mechanical capture. Use analgesia and sedation as needed.*

Figure 22.3: # Asystole treatment algorithm

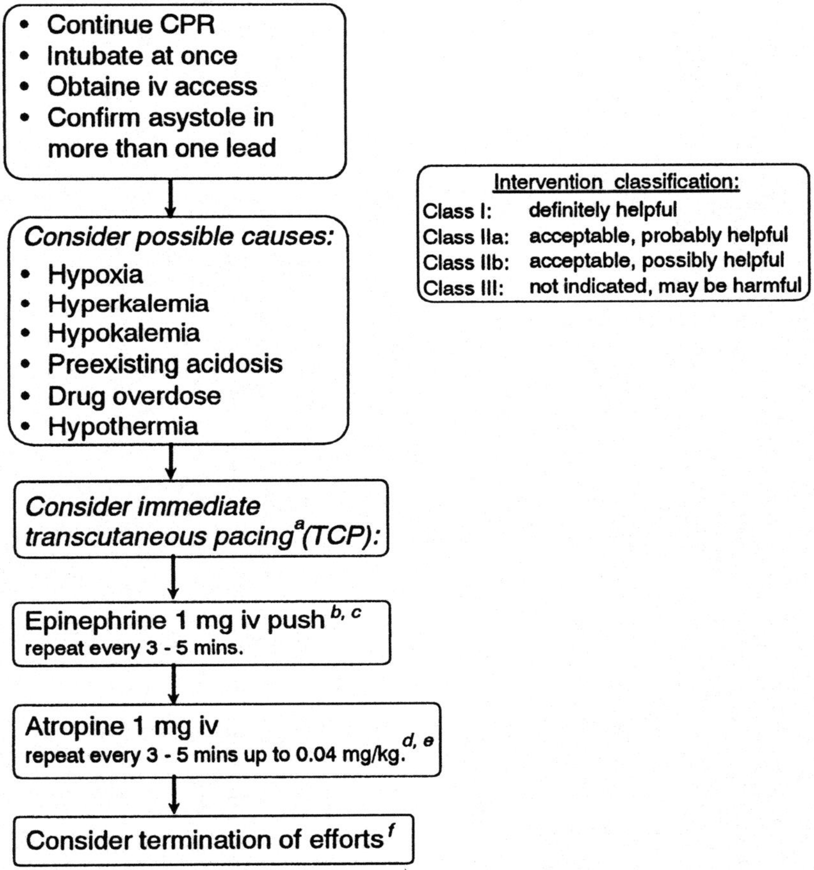

- Continue CPR
- Intubate at once
- Obtaine iv access
- Confirm asystole in
  more than one lead

Intervention classification:	
Class I:	definitely helpful
Class IIa:	acceptable, probably helpful
Class IIb:	acceptable, possibly helpful
Class III:	not indicated, may be harmful

Consider possible causes:

- Hypoxia
- Hyperkalemia
- Hypokalemia
- Preexisting acidosis
- Drug overdose
- Hypothermia

Consider immediate transcutaneous pacing[a] (TCP):

Epinephrine 1 mg iv push [b, c]
repeat every 3 - 5 mins.

Atropine 1 mg iv
repeat every 3 - 5 mins up to 0.04 mg/kg. [d, e]

Consider termination of efforts [f]

Footnotes for asystole algorithm:
a. *TCP is a class IIb intervention. Lack of success may be due to delays in pacing. To be effective TCP must be performed early, simultaneously with drugs. Evidence does not support routine use of TCP for asystole.*
b. *The recommended dose of epinephrine is 1 mg iv push every 3 - 5 mins. If this approach fails, several Class IIb dosing regimens can be considered: Intermediate epinephrine 2 - 5 mg iv push, every 3 - 5 min; Escalating epinephrine 1 mg - 3 mg - 5 mg iv push, 3 min apar;, High epinephrine 0.1 mg/kg iv push, every 3 - 5 min.*
c. *Sodium bicarbonate 1 mEq/kg is Class I if the patient has known perexisting hyperkalemia.*
d. *Shorter atropine dosing intervals are Class IIb in asystolic arrest.*
e. *Sodium bicarbonate 1 mEq/kg:*
   Class IIa: if known preexisting bicarbonate-responsive acidosis; if overdose with tricyclic antidepressants; to alkalinize the urine in drug overdoses.
   Class IIb: if intubated and continued long arrest interval; upon return of spontaneous circulation after long arrest interval. Class III: hypoxic lactic acidosis
f. *If patient remains in asystole or other agonal rhythms after successful intubation and initial medications and no reversible causes are identified, consider termination of resuscitative efforts by a physician.*
   Consider time interval since arrest.

Figure 22.4: Ventricular Fibrillation - Pulseless Ventricular Tachycardia Algorithm (VF / VT)

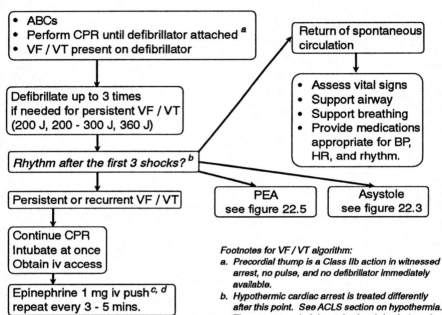

- ABCs
- Perform CPR until defibrillator attached [a]
- VF / VT present on defibrillator

Return of spontaneous circulation

Defibrillate up to 3 times if needed for persistent VF / VT (200 J, 200 - 300 J, 360 J)

- Assess vital signs
- Support airway
- Support breathing
- Provide medications appropriate for BP, HR, and rhythm.

Rhythm after the first 3 shocks? [b]

Persistent or recurrent VF / VT

PEA
see figure 22.5

Asystole
see figure 22.3

Continue CPR
Intubate at once
Obtain iv access

Epinephrine 1 mg iv push [c, d]
repeat every 3 - 5 mins.

Defibrillate 360 J within 30 - 60 secs [e]

Administer medications of probable benefit (Class IIa) in persistent or recurrent VF / VT [f, g]

Defibrillate 360 J, 30 - 60 secs after each dose of medication [e]
Pattern should be drug-shock, drug-shock

Footnotes for VF / VT algorithm:
a. *Precordial thump is a Class IIb action in witnessed arrest, no pulse, and no defibrillator immediately available.*
b. *Hypothermic cardiac arrest is treated differently after this point. See ACLS section on hypothermia.*
c. *The recommended dose of epinephrine is 1 mg iv push every 3 - 5 mins. If this approach fails, several Class IIb dosing regimens can be considered (see footnotes figure 22.3 b).*
d. *Sodium bicarbonate (1 mEq/kg) is Class I if patient has known preexisting hyperkalemia.*
e. *Multiple sequenced shocks (200 J, 200 - 300 J, 360 J) are acceptable here (Class I), especially when medications are delayed.*
f. *Medications:*
   Lidocaine 1.5 mg/kg iv push. Repeat in 3 - 5 mins to total loading dose of 3 mg/kg; then use Bretylium 5 mg/kg iv push. Repeat in 5 mins at 10 mg/kg
   Magnesium sulfate 1 - 2 gm iv in torsade de pointes or suspected hypomagnesemic state or severe refractory VF
   Procainamide 30 mg/min in refractory VF (maximum total 17 mg/kg).
g. *Sodium bicarbonate (1 mEq/kg iv):*
   (see footnotes figure 22.3 e)

Figure 22.5: Algorithm for
Pulseless Electrical Activity (PEA)
(Electromechanical Dissociation [EMD])

Includes:

- Electromechanical dissociation (EMD)
- Pseudo-EMD
- Idioventricular rhythms
- Ventricular escape rhythms
- Bradyasytolic rhythms
- Postdefibrillation idioventricular rhythms

- Continue CPR
- Intubate at once
- Obtain iv access
- Assess blood flow using doppler ultrasound

Consider possible causes
(parentheses = possible therapies and treatments)

- Hypovolemia (volume infusion)
- Hypoxia (ventilation)
- Cardiac tamponade (pericardiocentesis)
- Tension pneumothorax (needle decompression)
- Hypothermia (see ACLS hypothermia algorithm)
- Massive pulmonary embolism (surgery, thrombolytics)
- Drug overdoses such as tricyclics, digitalis, beta-blockers, calcium channel blockers
- Hyperkalemia [a]
- Acidosis [b]
- Massive acute myocardial infarction

Epinephrine 1 mg iv push [a, c]
repeat every 3 - 5 min.

If absolute bradycardia (< 60 beats/min) or
relative bradycardia, give atropine 1 mg iv
Repeat every 3 - 5 min to a total of 0.04 mg/kg. [d]

Footnotes for Pulseless Electrical Activity:
a. Sodium bicarbonate 1 mEq/kg is Class I if patient has known preexisting hyperkalemia
b. See footnote figure 22.3 e.
c. See footnote figure 22.3 b.
d. Shorter atropine dosing intervals are possibly helpful in cardiac arrest (Class IIb).

Table 22.3: Properties of cardiovascular drugs. (†† invasive pressure monitoring manditory)

Drug	Receptor Activity α-1 α-2 β-1 β-2	Single Bolus Dose	Infusion Rate and Preparation	Comments
Epinephrine †† (Adrenalin)	2+ 3+ 1+ 2+	Anaphylaxis: 3 - 5 mcg/kg Arrest: 1 mg	0.01 - 0.2 mcg/kg/min; 4 mg in 500 ml (8 mcg/ml)	Inotropic beta effects at 0.02 - 0.09 mcg/kg/min, pressor alpha effects at > 0.09 mcg/kg/min. Used for hypotension with myocardial depression.
Aminone †† (Inocor)	Phosphodiesterase inhibitor with positive inotropic action independent of adrenergic receptors.	0.75 mg/kg over 2 - 3 mins.	2 - 10 mcg/kg/min	CO increased, HR unchanged, BP may decrease. PAP, PCWP, SVR all decrease. Used as an inotrope in patients with end stage heart disease. Produces arterial and venous vasodilation and may decrease BP.
Dopamine †† (Inotropin)	1-4+ 0 1+ 2-4+ plus Dopamine receptor agonist		1 - 10 mcg/kg/min 400 mg in 500 ml (800 mcg/ml)	Renal effects via dopaminergic DA-1 receptor at 1 - 4 mcg/kg/min. At 5 - 10 mcg/kg/min beta effects predominate with an increase in HR, and CO. Above 10 mcg/kg/min alpha effects predominate and renal blood flow may decrease. Commonly used in lower doses to increase CO while preserving renal perfusion.
Dobutamine †† (Dobutrex)	0-1+ 0 1+ 3+		1 - 20 mcg/kg/min 500 mg in 500 ml (1 mg/ml)	CO increases, SVR and PCWP decrease. At lower doses CO increases without severe tachycardia or hypotension. At 10 - 15 mcg/kg/min, HR and vasodilation become more prominent. BP may not change. Used to increase CO.

Table 22.4: Properties of cardiovascular drugs. (^{tt}invasive pressure monitoring manditory)

Drug	Receptor Activity α-1	α-2	β-1	β-2	Single Bolus Dose	Infusion Rate and Preparation	Comments
Norepinephrine (Levophed)	4+	4+	2+	0		0.05 - 0.5 mcg/kg/min^{tt} 4 mg in 500 ml (8 mcg/ml)	Direct alpha and beta receptor agonist Decreases in renal blood flow occur with even low doses. At low doses the alpha effects increase blood pressure, causing vasoconstriction, and reflex bradycardia. At higher doses, beta receptor stimulation increases contractility.
Phenylephrine (Neosynephrine)	4+	0	1+	0	50 - 100 mcg	0.1 - 0.5 mcg/kg/min^{tt} 10 mg in 500 ml (20 mcg/ml)	Phenylephrine represents an almost pure alpha-1 agonist. Beta stimulation only occurs at very high doses. Phenylephrine may be used temporarily to provide profound vasoconstriction while the underlying cause of hypotension is corrected. Reflex bradycardia may occur. May be useful in patients with hypotension associated with a decreased SVR and tachycardia.
Ephedrine	3+	0	2+	1+	5 - 10 mg iv 25 - 50 mg im	Onset within 1 minute with a duration of 5 - 10 minutes. Generally not used as an infusion due to tachyphylaxis. (50 mg/ml amp)	Ephedrine is an indirect acting alpha and beta agonist. It causes vasoconstriction and an increase in heart rate, blood pressure and cardiac output. It is useful in patients with hypotension without tachycardia. It is the drug of choice for hypotension due to regional anaesthesia during labour and delivery as its combined adrenergic effects result in an increase in blood pressure without uterine vasoconstriction.

Table 22.5: Properties of cardiovascular drugs. (†† invasive pressure monitoring manditory)

Drug	Mechanism of Action	Single Bolus Dose	Infusion Rate and Preparation	Comments
Nitroprusside†† (Nipride)	Direct arterial and venous vasodilation	1 - 2 mcg/kg iv	0.2 - 8.0 mcg/kg/min. 50 mg in 500 ml (100 mcg/ml)	Useful in patients requiring minute to minute control of their blood pressure. A reflex tachycardia and increase in plasma renin levels may result from administration. Tachyphlaxis and cyanide toxicity may occur with infusions of greater than 6 mcg/kg/min for 2 or more hours.
Nitroglycerine (Nitrostat)	Direct venous vasodilation	0.3 - 0.6 mg SL 10 - 200 mcg iv	0.1 - 5.0 mcg/kg/min†† 50 mg in 500 ml (100 mcg/ml)	Direct venous vasodilation results in a reduction in preload and blood pressure. NTG improves LV performance and coronary blood flow. It is useful in treating congestive heart failure, coronary artery ischemia, and pulmonary hypertension.
Propranolol (Inderal)	Non-selective Beta-1 and Beta-2 Antagonist	0.25 - 1 mg iv	Maximum iv dose 10 mg. Not to exceed 3 mg iv every 5 minutes	Depresses heart rate, contractility, cardiac output and blood pressure. Potential side effects of beta antagonists include pulmonary edema, bronchoconstriction, coronary vasoconstriction, heart block, and impaired insulin release. It is useful in controlling tachycardia associated with coronary ischemia or hypertension.
Labetalol (Trandate)	4:1 Non-Selective Beta Antagonist to Alpha-1 Antagonist	0.05 - 0.25 mg/kg iv (5 - 20 mg iv over 2 mins)	2 amps (40 ml) with 160 ml NS (1 mg/ml) 2 mg/min.	Used in the treatment of hypertension and tachycardia. Reduces both blood pressure and heart rate. Labetalol has a relatively slow onset of 5 to 10 minutes, and can be used without direct arterial pressure monitoring.

Table 22.6: Properties of cardiovascular drugs.

Drug	Mechanism of Action	Single Bolus Dose	Comments
Calcium Chloride	No beta adrenergic activity. Rapid direct acting inotrope with a duration of 5 - 10 minutes.	1 - 10 mg/kg iv	Used to treat hypocalcemia, ECG changes of hypocalcemia in the presence of hypotension, and calcium channel blocker overdose. May also be useful in the treatment of hypermagnesemia, and to protect the myocardium from the effects of hyperkalemia.
Metoprolol (Betabloc)	Selective beta-1 antagonist	1 - 5 mg iv every 2 - 5 mins prn., may require up to 15 mg for full beta blockade.	Useful in controlling hypertension, tachycardia, and reducing myocardial ischemia. Potential side effects include bradycardia, heart block, pulmonary edema, bronchospasm, and impaired insulin release resulting in hypoglycemia.
Esmolol (Brevibloc)	Selective beta-1 antagonist	Single bolus: 0.5 mg/kg iv Infusion: 1 mg/ml solution 50 - 300 mcg/kg/min	Rapid onset of less than 2 minutes with a duration of less than 30 minutes. Indicated in the treatment of hypertension and tachycardia in patients at risk of hemodynamically induced myocardial ischemia. Also indicated in the control of the ventricular rate in acute atrial fibrillation and atrial flutter.
Verapamil (Isoptin)	Calcium channel antagonist	Single bolus: 2.5 - 5 mg iv maximum 10 mg iv.	Useful in terminating a supraventricular dysrhythmia. Also used in controlling the ventricular rate in patients with atrial fibrillation and atrial flutter. Contraindicated in pre-excitation syndromes (e.g., Wolff-Parkinson-White syndrome) as it may increase conduction in the accessory pathway.

Table 22.7: Properties of cardiovascular drugs.

Drug	Mechanism of Action	Single Bolus Dose	Comments
Atropine	Anticholinergic	0.3 - 0.6 mg iv increments max. 3 mg	Most commonly used to treat bradycardia (heart rate < 45 bpm). Also useful as an antisialogogue to dry oral secretions and aid oropharyngeal topical anaesthesia for an *awake* fiberoptic intubation.
Adenosine (Adenocard)	Antidysrhythmic	6 mg iv	Useful in paroxysmal supraventricular tachycardia's. May be associated with significant hypotension, facial flushing, and shortness of breath. Does not convert atrial fibrillation, atrial flutter, or ventricular tachycardia to a sinus rhythm, but may be useful in distinquishing an SVT from other tachydysrhythmias.
Enalapril (Vasotec)	Angiotensin converting enzyme inhibitor	1.25 mg iv maintenance 1.25 mg iv q6hrs.	Useful in treating hypertension and heart failure. Onset within 15 minutes, with maximum effect between 1 - 4 hours. Use with caution in patients with renal insufficiency. Decrease in BP is exagerated in patients on diuretics. Hypotension responds to volume expansion.
Nifedipine (Adalat)	Calcium channel blocker	10 mg sublingual Usual dose is 10 - 20 mg po tid Maximum dose is 120 mg per day.	Used in treating hypertension, coronary vasospasm, and angina. Especially useful in treating hypertension in the npo patient. Vasodilation is accompanied with a decrease in BP, SVR and an increase in HR. Negative inotropic action of nifedipine with beta blockers may precipitate heart failure. Nifedipine displaces digoxin and increases it's plasma level.

CHAPTER 23

Oxygen Therapy and Hypoxia

Oxygen is an essential and vital substrate used for many metabolic functions. Over 200 oxidase enzyme systems participate in our body's metabolic processes. The cytochrome c oxidase enzyme system in the mitochondria is responsible for over 90 percent of the bodies oxygen consumption. This enzyme system provides energy as adenosine triphosphate (ATP) for bodily functions through the oxidative phosphorylation of food products.

Under normal resting conditions, circulatory arrest with anoxia will result in brain cell injury within 1 minute and irreparable damage by 5 minutes. The heart, liver, kidney, and skeletal muscle have decreasing sensitivities to the effects of anoxia. Skeletal muscle is able to tolerate anoxic periods of up to two hours without suffering irreversible damage.

The Oxygen Cascade:

The partial pressure of oxygen is the concentration of oxygen multiplied by the barometric pressure. At one atmosphere of pressure, the partial pressure of oxygen is 160 mm Hg (760 mm Hg x 21% = 160 mm Hg). While the oxygen concentration on top of Mount Everest remains at 21% at an altitude of 26,000

feet, the barometric pressure is only 270 mm Hg. Hence the partial pressure of oxygen is only 47 mm Hg (270 mm Hg x 21% = 47 mm Hg).

The oxygen cascade refers to the progressive decrease in the partial pressure of oxygen from the ambient air to the tissue level (see figure 23.1). At sea level, the inspired partial pressure of

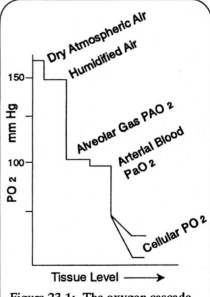

Figure 23.1: The oxygen cascade, illustrating the decreasing levels of PO_2 from the ambient air to the mitochondria.

Table 23.1: Factors influencing oxygenation at various levels in the oxygen cascade.

Partial Pressure	Affected by:	
I: Inspired Oxygen PiO_2	Barometric Pressure P_B	Oxygen Concentration FiO_2
II: Alveolar Gas PAO_2	Oxygen Consumption VO_2	Alveolar Ventilation V_A
III: Arterial Blood PaO_2	Dead Space Ventilation $\uparrow V/Q$	Shunt $\downarrow V/Q$
IV: Cellular PO_2	Cardiac Output CO	Hemoglobin Hb

oxygen is 160 mm Hg. At the tissue level, the partial pressure of oxygen in the mitochondria varies from 4 to 23 mm Hg. Hence, there is a progressive decrease in the partial pressure of oxygen from the alveolar and arterial level, to the cellular level. Table 23.1 lists various factors that influence the oxygen partial pressures at each level of the cascade.

I: A decrease in either the inspired oxygen concentration or the barometric pressure (e.g., in a high altitude environment) will lower the inspired oxygen partial pressure (FiO_2).

II: An increase in either oxygen consumption (e.g., as a consequence of sepsis or shivering) or a decrease in alveolar ventilation will decrease the alveolar oxygen partial pressure (PAO_2).

III: Arterial hypoxemia may occur as a result of ventilation perfusion abnormalities. These mismatches occur with an increase in either dead space ventilation or shunted blood.

IV: Tissue hypoxia will result whenever any of the above factors cause a decrease in the PiO_2, PAO_2, or PaO_2. In addition, tissue hypoxia results from either inadequate cardiac output (with poor tissue perfusion), or from an insufficient amount of hemoglobin to carry oxygen to the tissues.

Hypoxia is defined as a low level of oxygen in the air, blood, or tissues. *Hypoxemia* is a low level of oxygen in the blood. *Cyanosis* is a descriptive term used to describe the dark bluish or purplish coloration of the skin and mucous membranes accompanying hypoxemia. Cyanosis becomes evident when the reduced hemoglobin (deoxy-

Table 23.2: Oxygen delivery systems for spontaneously breathing patients.

O₂ Delivery Device	Flow Rate (L/min.)	Percent Oxygen
Nasal prongs	1 - 6	24 - 44% FiO_2 increases by approximately 4% for every 1L/min. increase in O_2 flow.
Simple face mask (Hudson mask)	5 - 6 6 - 7 7 - 8	40% 50% 60%
Venturi mask	4 - 12	24, 28, 31, 35, 40%
Non-rebreathing mask with reservoir bag.	6 7 8 9 - 10	60% 70% 80% 80% +
Puritan mask with: Single bottle setup Double bottle setup	> 10 L/min.	35 - 50% 50 - 80% +

hemoglobin) exceeds 5 grams per 100 ml of blood. It may be detected at an oxygen saturation as high as 85%, provided there is a normal hemoglobin level, good lighting conditions, and no excessive pigmentation. At an oxygen saturation of 75%, which corresponds to a PaO_2 of approximately 40 mm Hg, cyanosis is generally easily detected (see figure 10.4 oxygen dissociation curve). Anemia, poor lighting conditions, and dark pigmentation may mask cyanosis and the presence of hypoxemia.

Oxygen Therapy:
Postoperative surgical patients, patients with pneumonia, and patients with postoperative atelectasis are common candidates for supplemental oxygen therapy. These patients do not necessarily require mechanical ventilatory support (see criteria for ventilation; table 7.1). A general goal of oxygen therapy is to achieve an oxygen saturation of at least 90%. At our institution, the minimal acceptable saturation for post-surgical patients who are cared for in a non critical care setting, such as a hospital ward, is 92%.

There are a number of oxygen delivery systems available for providing supplemental oxygen to patients who are breathing spontaneously (table 23.2). Oxygen delivered by nasal prongs is

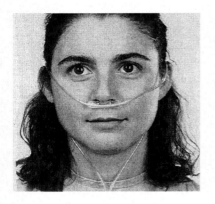

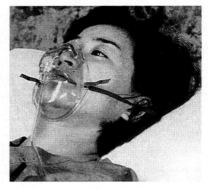

Nasal prongs

Simple face mask oxygen
(Hudson face mask)

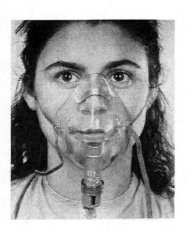

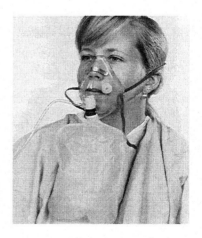

Venturi face mask

Non-rebreathing face mask
with reservoir bag.

Figure 23.2: Oxygen delivery systems for spontaneously breathing
patients.

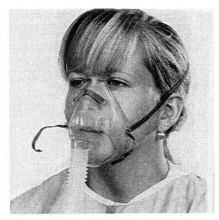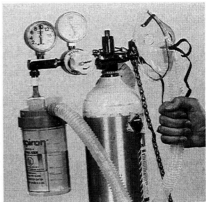

Figure. 23.3: The puritan face mask provides a high level humidity and predicatable concentrations of oxygen. Shown here with a single bottle set up for delivering inspired concentrations of up to 50%.

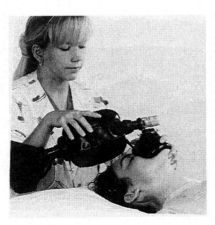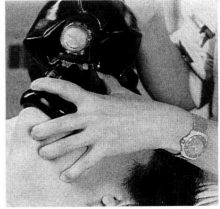

Figure 23.4: The Ambu manual resuscitation bag and mask unit. Used for providing primary airway management in patients requiring positive pressure ventilation and oxygenation. Note the hand and finger positioning on the mask. The fingers are used to displace the mandible forward and create a seal between the mask and the patient's face.

generally well tolerated, provided the flow rate is limited to less than 5 or 6 liters per minute. Flow rates above these levels cause an uncomfortable drying of the nasal mucosa. Common masks used to provide supplemental oxygen include the simple (Hudson) face mask, the venturi mask, and the non-rebreathing mask with reservoir bag. The type of mask utilized depends on the patient's tolerance, the desired inspired concentration of oxygen, the desired level of humidification, and economic considerations.

Entrainment of room air will result in a decrease in the inspired oxygen concentration. In general, the higher the patient's minute ventilation the greater will be the reduction in the inspired oxygen concentration. A simple face mask and nasal prongs are two examples of low flow oxygen delivery systems. These devices have a limited reservoir to store oxygen and are unable to deliver consistent inspired oxygen concentrations in the setting of varying respiratory rates and tidal volumes.

The venturi, non-rebreathing, and puritan face masks are high flow oxygen delivery systems. They are suitable for delivering consistent and predictable concentrations of oxygen (see figures 23.2 and 23.3). The venturi mask is designed to deliver specific percentages of oxygen by varying the size of the air entrainment port and the oxygen flow rate. A non-rebreathing mask with a reservoir bag allows high concentrations of oxygen to be delivered to a spontaneously breathing patient.

The puritan mask delivers the highest level of humidified oxygen of all these systems. When two outlet sources are connected to the puritan mask, oxygen flow rates of greater than 30 liters per minute can be achieved, ensuring a consistent inspired oxyen concentration by minimizing room air entrainment. One ought to use a double flow setup or a non-rebreathing face mask with reservoir bag, when greater than 50% inspired oxygen concentration is required.

A manual resuscitation unit, such as the Ambu bag and mask is used to provide positive pressure ventilation and oxygenation (figure 23.4). This can be used as the primary system for airway management in the patient requiring ventilatory support. Adequate oxygenation and ventilation can be maintained for prolonged periods of time while other supportive therapy is initiated. If tracheal intubation is required, mask ventilation should be maintained until all the equipment is available and properly checked. The mask should fit over the bridge of the nose, producing an air tight seal around the nose, cheeks, and chin. Change the size of mask, or insert an oral or nasal airway if you encounter difficulty maintaining airway patency or positive pressure ventilation.

Note the hand and finger positions used when providing positive pressure ventilation with an Ambu bag and mask unit (figure 23.4). The thumb is positioned over the nasal bridge of the mask. The index finger exerts downward pressure on the base of the mask over the chin.

The middle finger lifts the mandible forward into the base of the mask. The little finger is hooked around the angle of the mandible and displaces the mandible forward to create an open airway.

Causes of Hypoxemia:

Hypoxemia may result from a decrease in the inspired oxygen concentration, a decrease in the minute ventilation, an increase in shunted blood, or a decrease

Table 23.3:	Causes of Hypoxemia
Decreased FiO_2	Decreased inspired oxygen concentration Decreased barometric pressure (high altitude)
Decreased alveolar ventilation	Hypoventilation - hypoventilation secondary to sedative drugs or pain are common causes.
Increased dead space ventilation (ventilation - perfusion inequality)	Unlike hypoxemia from shunted blood, hypoxemia from V/Q inequalities responds to supplemental oxygen therapy. - conditions which increase zone I in the lung will result in an increase in dead space ventilation. Examples include hypovolemia, and high airway pressures with positive pressure ventilation. Other examples of dead space ventilation include pulmonary embolism, emphysema, and bronchitis.
Increased shunt	Perfusion of alveoli without ventilation results in an intrapulmonary shunting of blood. Examples include atelectasis, aspiration, congestive heart failure, pneumonia, and endobronchial intubation with lobar collapse. Shunting of blood may also occur outside the lung as a result of intracardiac shunts, or peripheral arteriovenous shunts.
Decreased diffusion	Problems with oxygen diffusing across the alveolar capillary membrane are rare, but may occur with high altitude, anemia, or severe exercise in normal individuals. Pulmonary fibrosis, emphysema, and interstitial pulmonary pathology such as sarcoidosis, may also result in a decrease in diffusion of oxygen and hypoxemia.

Table 23.4:	Causes of Tissue Hypoxia
Decreased functional hemoglobin	Anemia, hemoglobinopathies
Decreased PaO$_2$	Hypoxemia (see table 23.3)
Decreased tissue perfusion	Shock states (see table 21.5) - hypovolemic - cardiogenic - distributive - obstructive
Cellular hypoxia	Histotoxic hypoxia - cyanide poisoning

in the diffusion of oxygen across the alveolar capillary membrane (see Table 23.3).

Tissue hypoxia will result from a decrease in circulating hemoglobin, a decrease in the arterial oxygen tension (PaO$_2$), a decrease in tissue perfusion, or from a cellular toxin such as cyanide (see Table 23.4).

References:

1. Shapiro BA., et.al: Oxygen therapy. Clinical application of respiratory care, 4th ed. Mosby year book. 1991; pp. 123 - 150.

2. Finucane BT, Santora AH. Airway management equipment. Principles of airway management. FA Davis Co. Philadelphia. 1988; pp. 34 - 68.

3. Barash PG, Cullen BF, Stoelting RK. Monitoring the anesthetized patient. Clinical anesthesia. Second edit. JB Lippincott Co. Philadelphia, 1993.

4. Nunn JF. Oxygen. Applied respiratory physiology. Third edit. Butterworth and Co. 1987; pp. 235 - 383.

Notes:

CHAPTER 24

Unusual Anaesthetic Complications

GREGORY ALLEN M.D., FRCPC AND GORDON REID M.D., FRCPC

In this chapter we shall present three life threatening anaesthetic related complications.

I. Malignant Hyperthermia (MH)

What is MH*?

Malignant hyperthermia is a rare clinical syndrome that has been observed during general anaesthesia. Patients may experience an acute fulminant form, which can be triggered by certain anaesthetic drugs, and result in a hypermetabolic state because of acute uncontrolled skeletal muscle metabolism. Rapid increases in oxygen consumption, carbon dioxide production and heat result in desaturation or cyanosis, elevated end-tidal CO_2 values and rapid increases in temperature (up to $1°C$ / 5 min), as well as a host of other abnormalities (see table 24.1).

How serious is it?

The mortality of MH has decreased from over 80% in the 1960's to less than 10%. Only about 10% of MH episodes are fulminant, with a rapid onset and severe physiological derangements and complications.

Table 24.1: Clinical features of malignant hyperthermia.

Hypermetabolism:
- Increased oxygen consumption
- Dark blood in surgical wound
- Cyanosis
- Increased CO_2 production
- Increased end-tidal CO_2
- Respiratory acidosis
- Elevated temperature
- Sweating
- Metabolic acidosis
- Increased lactate levels
- Tachycardia
- Tachypnea
- Arrhythmias
- Unstable BP

Muscle Rigidity:
- Masseter muscle spasm (unable to open mouth)
- Chest wall rigidity (difficulty ventilating)
- Abdominal rigidity
- Limb rigidity

Rhabdomyolysis:
- Hyperkalemia
- Painful, tender, swollen muscles
- Elevated creatinine kinase (CPK)
- Myoglobinemia, myoglobinuria

Can you predict who is susceptible?
MH is an inherited disorder of skeletal muscle. History and physical examination are usually not helpful in the preoperative diagnosis of MH-susceptibility. A history of uneventful anaesthetics in the past is no guarantee that the patient does not have the disorder. A history of intraoperative cardiac arrest, muscle rigidity or stiffness under anaesthesia, high fever under anaesthesia, dark urine after anaesthesia, or family member who died unexpectedly under anaesthesia warrant further investigations and a review of any available medical records. Patients with muscular dystrophy or myopathy have been observed to have an increased association with MH.

The pattern of inheritance is autosomal dominant. Molecular geneticists have identified an abnormal locus on chromosome 19q in the area of the skeletal muscle ryanodine receptor (RYR 1). The ryanodine receptor is associated with the calcium influx channel in the skeletal muscle sarcoplasmic reticulum, and is thought to be the site of the MH defect. Unfortunately a simple screening blood test is not likely to be available in the near future because of the complicated genetics. The only test currently used to make the diagnosis reliably and accurately involves taking a muscle biopsy from the patient's quadriceps muscle. Muscle from a patient with MH is noted to develop an abnormally strong response when exposed to caffeine or halothane. The test is only done at certain special testing centres, and is not used for screening patients.

What anaesthetic agents trigger MH*?
The triggers of MH include the depolarizing muscle relaxant succinylcholine, and any of the volatile anaesthetic agents (isoflurane, halothane, enflurane, and sevoflurane).

What anaesthetic agents are safe?
Intravenous agents including any barbiturate (eg. pentothal), benzodiazepine (eg. midazolam, diazepam), as well as propofol or ketamine may be used safely to induce and/or maintain anaesthesia. Nitrous oxide and any narcotic may be used. Muscle relaxants such as pancuronium, vecuronium or atracurium can all be used, and their action reversed with a combination of an anticholinesterase and anticholinergic agents such as neostigmine and glycopyrrolate, or edrophonium and atropine. Local anaesthetic agents including the amide class (e.g., bupivicaine, lidocaine), and ester class (e.g., tetracaine, chlorprocaine), with or without epinephrine, have been used safely in MH patients.

How do you treat an MH crisis?
Early diagnosis and administration of dantrolene are the primary focus of treating and reversing the hypermetabolic abnormalities of MH. Measures such as cooling, treating hyperkalemia, arrhythmias, etc., focus on dealing with the consequences of the MH reaction. Dantrolene is classified as a skeletal muscle relaxant, and is used occasionally in patients with disorders of skeletal muscle spasticity. It may result in skeletal muscle weakness, but typically does not result in muscle paralysis. It is supplied as a yellow powder in vials containing 20 mg of dantrolene and 3

grams of mannitol. Each vial of dantrolene is mixed with 60 mL of water, which can be a time consuming task because dantrolene is so insoluble. Every hospital that provides general anaesthetic services is required to keep a current stock (minimum 36 vials) of dantrolene available in their pharmacy department.

Table 24.2: Treatment of a suspected MH crisis.
Malignant Hyperthermia Association guidelines (Revised 1993).

1. Immediately discontinue volatile anaesthetic agent and succinylcholine. Hyperventilate with 100% oxygen at high flow rates (> 10 L/min).

2. Administer dantrolene sodium 2 - 3 mg/kg initial bolus, up to 10 mg/kg.

3. Administer bicarbonate to correct metabolic acidosis as guided by blood gas analysis. In the absence of blood gas analysis, 1 - 2 mg/kg should be administered.

4. At the same time institute cooling measures for the hyperthermic patient, (goal = 38°C). Administer iced saline 15 mL/kg iv q 15 minutes x 3.
   a. Lavage stomach, bladder, rectum and open cavities with iced saline as appropriate.
   b. Surface cool with ice and hypothermia blanket.
   c. Monitor closely since over-vigorous treatment may lead to hypothermia.

5. Dysrhythmias will usually respond to treatment of acidosis and hyperkalemia. Persistent dysrhythmias may be treated as per ACLS protocol, with the exception of calcium channel blockers (calcium channel blockers in these patients may result in hyperkalemia and cardiovascular collapse).

6. Determine and monitor end-tidal CO_2, arterial, central or femoral venous blood gases, serum potassium, calcium, clotting studies and urine output.

7. Hyperkalemia is common and should be treated with hyperventilation, bicarbonate, intravenous glucose and insulin (10 units regular insulin in 50 mL 50% glucose titrated to potassium level). Life-threatening hyperkalemia may also be treated with calcium administration (eg. 2 - 5 mg/kg of $CaCl_2$).

8. Ensure urine output of greater than 2 mL/kg/hr. Consider central venous or PA monitoring because of fluid shifts and hemodynamic instability that may occur.

9. Boys less than 9 years of age who experience sudden cardiac arrest after succinylcholine in the absence of hypoxemia should be treated for acute hyperkalemia first. In this situation, calcium chloride should be administered along with other means to reduce serum potassium. They should be presumed to have subclinical muscular dystrophy.

Source: Malignant Hyperthermia Association of the United States, Westport, CT, USA

Potential complications of MH include:

• Acute hyperkalemia (from cell lysis)
• Acute renal failure (myoglobinuria)
• Arrhythmias
• Pulmonary edema
• ARDS
• Severe muscle pains, weakness
• Hepatic dysfunction
• Hemolysis
• Disseminated intravascular coagulation
• Cerebral injury - seizures, coma

Following the initial treatment of an MH suspected crisis:

A. The patient should be observed in an ICU setting for at least 24 hours, since recrudescence of MH may occur, particularly following a fulminant case.

B. Administer dantrolene 1 mg/kg iv every 6 hours for 24 - 48 hours after the episode.

C. Follow ABG, CPK, potassium, calcium, urine and serum myoglobin, clotting studies and core body temperature until such time as they return to normal values (eg. 6 hours). Central temperature (eg. rectal, esophageal) should be continuously monitored until stable.

D. Counsel the patient and family regarding MH and further precautions. Refer the patient to the MH North American registry, and biopsy centre.

MH related issues:

Postoperative fever:
An increase in body temperature above 38.5°C in the perioperative period is the result of either (1) an increase in body heat production, (2) a decrease in body heat elimination, or (3) the result of active warming measures. Postoperative fevers are very rarely due to MH. More common causes of an elevated temperature in the perioperative period include:

• coexisting infections
• anticholinergic medications (e.g., atropine resulting in decreased sweating)
• transfusion reaction
• dehydration
• excessive coverings on the patient
• elevated room temperature
• active warming measures (blankets, fluids)
• thyrotoxicosis

Heat stroke:
MH patients may be more susceptible to heat stroke compared to the normal population. However, most patients suffering from heat stroke are not MH susceptible. Patients who have suffered from heat stroke and also have an abnormal family history of anaesthesia problems suggestive of MH, should be investigated for MH.

II: Aspiration Syndrome.

Chapter nine introduced the concept of a rapid sequence induction and identified factors that placed a patient at risk for gastric aspiration. The severity of gastric aspiration is related to the volume and acidity of the aspirate, the presence of contaminated particulate matter (e.g., bowel contents) and the former health of the patient.

Strategies useful in reducing the perioperative risk of gastric aspiration include*:

1. *Avoid impairing airway reflexes.* The risk of gastric aspiration is reduced in the awake patient. Surgery that can be accomplished with local or regional anaesthesia should be considered in the patient at risk of aspiration.

2. *Reduce gastric volume and acidity.* A period of fasting (minimal 8 hours for solid foods and 4 hours for clear liquids) is mandatory in a patient undergoing non-emergency surgery. A planned regional or local anaesthetic does not negate the need to fast as unforseen events may arise necessitating a general anaesthetic. Metochlorpropamide and domperidone have been used to stimulate gastric motility and promote gastric emptying. H-2 antagonists and antacids are useful when given preoperatively to reduce both gastric secretion and acidity. Sodium citrate is the antacid of choice in anaesthesia as it is non-particulate and produces the least damage of

any antacid if aspirated. Gastric emptying by nasogastric tube is important in patients with a bowel obstruction.

3. In patients with an anticipated difficult intubation, topicalization and local anaesthetic blocks of the upper airway will permit the trachea to be intubated with the patient awake. This reduces the chance of a failed intubation, difficult mask ventilation, and subsequent gastric aspiration.

4. Patients with identified risk factors for gastric aspiration who require general anaesthesia (see Table 9.1), must have a rapid sequence induction. This involves a period of preoxygenation, the application of cricoid pressure, and tracheal intubation with a cuffed ETT (see chapter 9; Rapid Sequence Induction). Extubation should only be performed when the following criteria are met:

a. the patient is responding to verbal commands
b. the patient has regained an oropharyngeal *gag* reflex
c. the patient is positioned on their side, and
d. the need for tracheal intubation is no longer present.

The consequences of gastric aspiration:

Apiration of a liquid causes a vigorous cough, accompanied by a transient period of hypoxemia in the normal awake adult. Significant cellular damage occurs in a dog model when the pH is less than 2.5 and the volume is greater than 0.4 ml/kg. If the liquid has a pH of 2.5 or more, it will generally not cause cellular damage. When gastric acid is aspirated, surfactant is destroyed, the alveoli collapse, and hemorrhage and exudation into the alveoli and interstitium occurs. Severe bronchospasm usually accompanies a significant aspiration. Lung compliance decreases as alveoli collapse, and areas of shunt occur, resulting in severe hypoxemia.

Aspiration of particulate (food or fecal) matter may result in blockage of distal bronchi, resulting in large areas of collapse, edema formation and shunting. Within the first few days a mononuclear foreign body response occurs. The lung distal to the obstructed bronchi collapses and fills with secretions. Without resolution, lung infection or abscess formation are inevitable.

Diagnosis of aspiration:

Early diagnosis and treatment may reduce the severity of the aspiration syndrome. During mask anaesthesia with either a face or laryngeal mask, the detection of aspiration may be difficult. Sudden laryngospasm, coughing or stridor may be the first indication that aspiration has occurred. Bronchospasm may also occur, and the compliance of the chest may decrease resulting in increased airway pressures during mechanical ventilation. Alternatively, desaturation with hypoxemia and the need for higher concentrations of oxygen may

be the only indication of aspiration. Gastric contents in the upper airway and mouth, may or may not, accompany gastric aspiration.

Treatment of aspiration:

The first few minutes following an aspiration are critical, and attempts must be made to remove as much material as possible from the mouth, pharynx and trachea. As the most common site for aspiration is the apical posterior segment of the right lung, the patient should be positioned head down in the right lateral position to limit spread to the left lung, and aid drainage by gravity. Immediate bronchoscopy is used to remove any particulate matter that has been aspirated.

With a significant aspiration, severe hypoxemia with decreased lung compliance and difficulty providing positive pressure ventilation are expected to occur within the first 30 to 60 minutes. Positive pressure ventilation with continuous positive airway pressure (CPAP) or positive end expiratory pressure (PEEP) are used to prevent alveolar collapse, limit the reduction in residual volume, and prevent further atelectasis and shunting. Crystalloid solutions are preferable to colloid solutions (see chapter 20), because the pulmonary capillary membrane is injured, and may allow colloid solutions to cross into the alveoli, increasing the degree of pulmonary edema.

Steroids are not generally indicated, and may promote granuloma formation in cases of aspirated food particles. Antibiotics are also not indicated, unless there is evidence of gross aspiration from bowel contents. Bronchodilators are used in treating bronchospasm. Prolonged positive pressure ventilation and critical management of intravascular volume status, oxygenation, and ventilation are the principles of treating a significant aspiration. Invasive monitoring and frequent blood gas analysis may be required. Mortality and morbidity usually results from the initial severe hypoxemia that occurs at the time of aspiration. This emphasizes the need for initial aggressive treatment.

III: Allergic reactions

Muscle relaxants and exposure to latex materials are the two most common causes of an allergic reaction occurring during anaesthesia. The frequency of anaphylactic shock is 1 in 3500 anaesthetics. The allergic response manifests within minutes of an intravenous injection of the offending agent. By contrast, signs of an allergic response resulting from latex are delayed.

Definitions:

Anaphylactoid is a general term used to describe the clinical features of an allergic reaction. The term anaphylactoid shock is used to designate an allergic reaction in which the mechanism may be either the result of a direct release of histamine, or from an immune mediated mechanism.

Anaphylactic or *anaphylaxis* is used when an allergic reaction is immune mediated, and implicates IgE antibodies and prior sensitization from previous

exposure to the drug. This form of reaction can be diagnosed with skin tests and specific antibody assays.

An *anaphylactoid reaction* occurs when the allergen causes direct release of histamine. This reaction is not immune mediated and IgE antibodies are not involved.

Table 24.3: Clinical Features*
• Anxiety, headache, nausea
• Impending sense of doom
• Dyspnea, tachypnea
• Tachycardia
• Flushing, hives, urticaria (70%)
• Facial, orbital, mucous membrane edema, sneezing
• Hoarseness, laryngeal edema
• Hypotension (85%)
• Bronchospasm (35%)
• Hypoxemia
• Desaturation
• Increased airway pressures

Table 24.3 lists the clinical manifestations of an allergic reaction. Exposure to the allergen results in the release of histamine, tryptase, leukotrienes and cytokines from mast cells and basophils. These act on both histamine (H1 and H2) receptors throughout the body producing the clinical features. An immediate brief surge in plasma histamine levels occurs followed by a gradual rise in tryptase levels which are specific to anaphylactic reactions and can be measured in the serum (see figure 24.1). Analysis of the urine can be used to detect a metabolite of histamine, urinary

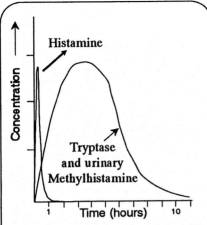

Figure 24.1: Schematic time profile of the release of histamine, tryptase, and urinary methylhistamine following anaphylaxis.

methylhistamine, and aid in the diagnosis. Elevated levels of urinary methylhistamine and serum tryptase support the diagnosis of an anaphylactic reaction, but do not identify the allergen. Serum IgE antibodies can be used to perform radioimmunoassays (RIAs) to identify the responsible allergen. Specific antibodies to thiopental, propofol, muscle relaxants and latex are now available. Blood and urine samples should be taken at 1 to 3 hours, and 24 hours after the reaction to measure these mediators. The patient should be referred for skin testing with cutaneous skin prick tests within two months of the reaction.

Muscle relaxants account for 70% of the cases of anaphylaxis during anaesthesia. The tertiary or quaternary ammonium group on muscle relaxants is frequently the antigenic site. As this is common to many muscle relaxants, cross reactivity between different relaxants is common. Prior exposure to a muscle relaxant is not required, as previous sensitization may have occurred following exposure to household products containing substances with ammonium structures (e.g., disinfectants, cosmetics). Latex allergy accounts for approximately 12% of allergic reactions. Patients with repeat exposure to latex products have an increased risk of a latex allergy. These include patients requiring repeat urinary catheterization (paraplegia, spina bifida), and health care workers who frequently work with latex gloves. Less than 15% of allergic reactions are the result of exposure to blood products, opioids, benzodiazepines, and antibiotics.

*Treatment of anaphylaxis:***

A useful memory tool in recalling the emergency treatment steps for anaphylaxis is to recall the *"Anaphylaxis ABCs"* :

A   Airway, and adrenaline
B   Breathing and benadryl
C   Crystalloids and cimetidine
s   steroids

Tachycardia with an allergic reaction results from the chronotropic effects of H2 receptor stimulation. Epinephrine is the principle initial drug treatment. In cases of severe hypotension or laryngospasm, 0.1 ml of 1:1000 epinephrine may be given intravenously, and repeated as needed. A single bolus dose of epinephrine should generally not exceed 0.5 ml (0.5 mg). Excessive epinephrine administration risks malignant arrhythmias (ventricular tachycardia, and ventricular fibrillation) severe hypertension, pulmonary edema, myocardial infarction and stroke. Nevertheless, patients taking beta-blockers may be resistant to the effects of epinephrine, and may require higher doses of epinephrine. The administration of beta- blockers, to control the heart rate response, is contraindicated in patients experiencing an anaphylactoid reaction.

Table 24.4: Management of Anaphylaxis during Anaesthesia

- Stop drug or allergen administration
- Provide 100% oxygen
- Discontinue surgery and anaesthesia as soon as feasible.
- Give epinephrine 50 - 100 mcg iv with hypotension, 0.5 - 1.0 mg iv with cardiovascular collapse.
- Epinephrine infusion 0.05 - 0.2 mcg/kg/min (see chapter 22).
- Crystalloids (e.g., NS, RL) iv, may require 2 - 4 liters for a 70 kg adult, i.e., 25 - 50 ml/kg.
- Diphenhydramine 50 mg iv (Benadryl® ~ 1 mg/kg)
- Cimetidine 300 mg iv, or ranitidine 50 mg iv
- Hydrocortisone 100 mg iv (Solucortef® ~ 1.5 mg/kg), or methylprednisolone (Solumedrol®) 1 mg/kg iv q6hrs x 24 hours.
- Inhaled salbutamol (ventolin®) for bronchospasm.
- Avoid beta blockers.

References:

1. Allen GC. Malignant Hyperthermia. *Aether* 1994; 1: 3 - 6.

2. Gibbs CP, Modell JH. Management of Aspiration Pneumonitis, Anesthesia 3rd edition. Edited by Miller RD. Churchill Livingstone Inc. 1990. pp. 1293 - 1319.

3. Laxenaire MC, Moneret-Vautrin DA. Allergy and Anaesthesia. *Aether* 1994; 2: 14 - 17.

Notes:

Appendix:

Intravenous Access

Intravenous (iv) cannulation provides direct access to the venous circulation. This discussion will focus on practical aspects of securing venous access to the peripheral circulation. Students are not expected to acquire skills for insertion of catheters into the central circulation, or for performing a venous cutdown during this rotation. Intravenous catheterization is most commonly indicated for administering medications or fluids, or to sample blood for analysis.

A plastic catheter, which is inserted over a hollow needle, is the most common intravenous catheter system used for peripheral venous cannulation. The length of the catheter, and it's internal diameter, the viscosity of the intravenous fluid, and the pressure differential between the vein and the fluid being administered all determine the maximum flow rate, as specified by the Hagen-Poiseuille equation:

Hagen-Poiseuille equation:

Flow $\propto \dfrac{\pi P r^4}{8nl}$

P = *pressure across the catheter*
r = *radius of the catheter*
n = *viscosity of the fluid*
l = *length of the catheter*

The Hagen-Poiseuille equation explains why a 5 inch long 16 gauge central venous catheter will achieve less than half the maximum flow rate of a 2 inch long 16 gauge peripheral catheter. Alternatively, by halving the radius of the catheter, the maximum flow rate will decrease to 1/16. Warming the intravenous fluids will cause venodilation, decrease fluid viscosity, and increase the maximum flow rate. Similarly, pressurizing the fluid in the intravenous bag will increase the pressure differential between the fluid and venous system and permit more rapid fluid administration.

Venous Anatomy:

The upper extremities venous anatomy is relatively consistent. Digital veins run proximally from the digits to the dorsal arch of veins on the dorsal surface of the hands. A vein can usually be located just above the head of the 3rd and 4th metacarpals. The dorsal arch turns radially to the anatomical snuff box, where a large superficial vein can be located at the level of the distal radial tubercle. This vein continues along the lateral forearm to the anticubital fossa where it joins other veins to form the cephalic vein. The cephalic vein can sometimes be followed up the arm over the biceps muscle, crossing the deltoid muscle anteriorly, and disappearing between the heads of the deltoid and pectoralis muscles to enter the axillary vein. Other superficial veins travel up the forearm to form the basilic vein located just medial to the insertion of the biceps muscle in the anticubital fossa. The basilic vein continues proximally (becoming obscured in the lower 1/3 of the arm as it enters the muscles of the arm) to join the axillary vein in the axilla. Identification of superficial veins may be difficult in obese patients. Fortunately, the volar aspect of the wrist generally lacks adipose tissue. Examination of this area may reveal small veins that can be used for access when attempts at other sites have failed.

The upper extremity is used for venous cannulation in the vast majority of patients. Patient anxiety (increased catecholamines), a cold environment (venoconstriction), adipose tissue, or a pre-existing fluid deficit, may make the identification of suitable veins for venous cannulation difficult. To improve the chance of successful cannulation, keep the extremity below the level of the heart, use a tourniquet around the biceps muscle to distend the vein, avoid cooling the patient, and consider using warm blankets or heating pads on the extremity to dilate the veins. When venous cannulation of the upper extremity fails, one can use the lower extremity. The foot has a dorsal venous arch that can be used for venous access. The saphenous vein is the equivalent to the superficial radial vein in the forearm. It continues from the dorsal arch of the foot to pass over the anterior aspect of the medial malleolus. It then travels up to the medial aspect of

the knee, passing behind the femoral condyle. It continues proximally along the medial thigh entering the thigh muscles approximately 1.5" below the inguinal ligament, where it joins the femoral vein. The anatomy of the femoral vessels (lateral to medial) can be recalled using the pneumonic **NAVEL**★ where:

N = Nerve
A = Artery
V = Vein
E = Empty space
L = Lymphatics

(★recall that the NAVEL pneumonic was also used for drugs which can be given through a tracheal tube. See pg. 50).

The femoral artery is located at the midpoint between the anterior superior iliac spine and the pubic symphysis. The femoral vein lies approximately 1 cm medial to the artery. Cannulation of the femoral vein is less popular than other veins because of the restriction in patient mobility, and the risks of infection or thrombosis. Peripheral intravenous catheters are generally too short to be used for the femoral vein, and a longer central venous catheter (approximately 5 inches in length) is more suitable.

Choice of site for intravenous cannulation:

The most common sites used for iv cannulation are the dorsum of the hand, medial aspect of the forearm, and the anticubital fossa. Of these, the dorsum of the hand is perhaps the most com-

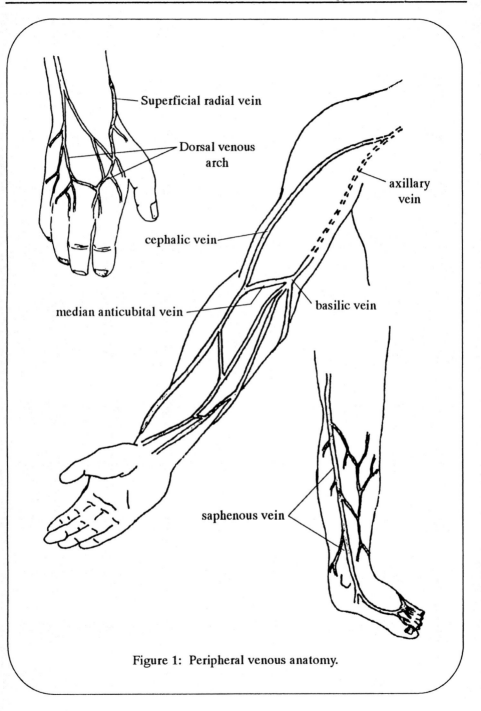

Figure 1: Peripheral venous anatomy.

mon choice. It allows one easy access to the vein, and, should the intravenous fail, one may still use a more proximal site. For patients who will require their intravenous for a period of time greater than 24 hours, the forearm may be a better choice. It restricts their activities less, and remains relatively immobile when they move their arms. They are also less likely to catch their intravenous on other objects.

The anticubital fossa is a good choice when a large vein is required, and the anticipated period in which the catheter will be used is a short one. As a general rule, however, it is best to chose a site for the intravenous that does not lie over a joint. When a patient flexes and extends their joint, the intravenous site will be uncomfortable, and this motion may dislodge the catheter from the vein making it interstitial. One also risks injuring the median nerve or catheterizing the brachial artery when attempting anticubital vein cannulation.

The lower extremity and femoral veins are less commonly chosen for iv access because they restrict patient's mobility and increase the risk of complications including infection, phlebitis, and thromboembolism.

Choice of Intravenous Size:

Intravenous catheters are supplied in various sizes and lengths. The size of catheter increases as the gauge number of the catheter decreases. In adult anaesthesia, we consider a 20 gauge catheter to be small. The catheters come in even numbers i.e., 14, 16, 18, 20, 22, 24, and 26 gauge catheters. The 24 and 26 gauge catheters are generally only used in the neonatal or paediatric population. Sixteen to 20 gauge catheters are the most common sizes used in adults. Catheter lengths for peripheral veins vary from 1" to 2".

Patients who may require blood products and large amounts of intravenous fluids should have several large bore intravenous catheters (i.e., 14 or 16 gauge). We routinely manage patients undergoing minor procedures, in which the need for rapid fluid administration is remote, with a single 18 or 20 gauge intravenous catheter.

Intravenous catheters of 18 gauge or larger may cause moderate discomfort when inserted in the awake patient. By using local anaesthesia, you may be able to decrease this discomfort. A 25 or 27 gauge needle can be used to administer approximately 1/4 ml of 2% lidocaine into the dermis either directly over the vein or immediately lateral to the vein. Aspiration before injection is not necessary. Insert the intravenous cannula <u>through</u> the local anaesthetic wheal.

Technique of Intravenous Cannulation:

Assemble your required equipment including: iv bag and tubing, iv catheters, tourniquet, alcohol swab, gloves, tape, (+/- povidone-iodine swab, 1/4 ml 2% lidocaine local anaesthetic in a 3 ml syringe with a 25 or 27 gauge needle, and gauze to clean spilt blood).

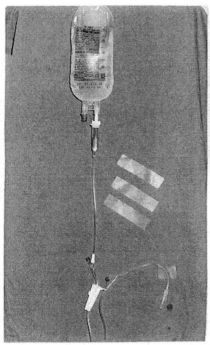

Intravenous bag, tubing and tape.

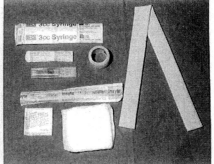

3 cc syringe, 2% lidocaine, 27 gauge needle, intravenous catheter, tape, tourniquet, and gauze.

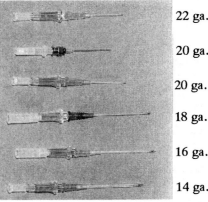

22 ga.

20 ga.

20 ga.

18 ga.

16 ga.

14 ga.

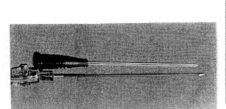

Intravenous catheter and needle. Note that the needle is longer than the catheter.

Common intravenous cannulas. Small bore = 22 and 20 gauge, Large bore = 16 and 14 gauge.

Figure 2: Equipment for peripheral intravenous access.

1. Apply a tourniquet to the extremity.
2. Identify a suitable vein. <u>Gently</u> tap over the vein to facilitate veno-dilation.
3. Cleanse the area with an alcohol swab (or povidone-iodine swab followed by an alcohol swab).
4. Wear disposable gloves (recommended).
5. *Optional:* Inject local anaesthesia with a 25 or 27 gauge needle into the dermis either directly over the vein or 2 - 3 mm lateral to it using 1/4 ml of 2% lidocaine.
6. *Optional:* Break the seal between the catheter and the needle (this may make it easier to advance the catheter off the needle once you enter the vein).
7. Immobilize the vein by applying traction to the skin distal to the insertion site with the hand that is not holding the intravenous catheter. Maintain immobilization of the vein during iv insertion. Avoid putting your hand immediately below the vein as this will prevent you from lowering the intravenous catheter into the same plane as the vein.
8. Hold the hub of the needle between your thumb and forefinger with the bevel facing up. Watch for the blood to flash back into the plastic hub when you enter the vein.
9. Puncture the skin <u>through</u> the an-aesthetic skin wheal holding the needle at a 30 - 45 degree angle to the vein. Advance the needle until the catheter is beneath the skin.
10. Lower the angle of the intravenous catheter to approximate that of the vein you are attempting to enter.
11. Advance the catheter and needle (maintaining skin traction and vein immobilization) visualizing where the tip of the needle is in relation to the vein, watching for a flash of blood in the hub of the catheter.
12. When blood comes back into the hub, advance the needle and cathe-ter another 2 mm to ensure the catheter is in the vein (and not still outside the wall of the vein).
13. Without moving the catheter, with-draw the needle approximately 1 cm. (Alternatively, without moving the needle, the catheter can be advanced over the tip of the needle by approximately 1 cm).
14. With the needle back from the tip of the catheter, advance both the needle and catheter together until you feel resistance or the catheter is fully inserted.
15. Release the tourniquet.
16. Using the hand that was maintaining skin traction, occlude the vein by pressing with your finger proximal to the tip of the catheter (lying in the vein). This prevents blood from coming back out of the catheter when the needle is removed.
17. Remove the needle, leaving the catheter in the vein.
18. Secure the intravenous tubing to the catheter (a luer lock connecting end accompanies certain iv tubing sys-tems).
19. Open the intravenous roller clamp, and adjust the flow to the desired rate.
20. Secure the intravenous to the patient with tape.

Figure 3: Venous anatomy, immobilization and cannulation.

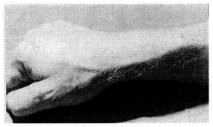

Superficial radial vein.

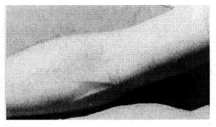

Basilic vein.

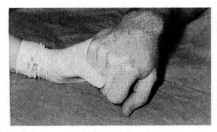

Immobilization of the dorsal
veins of the hand.

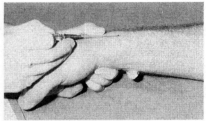

Immobilization of the
superficial radial vein.

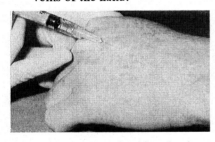

Local anaesthetic skin wheal.

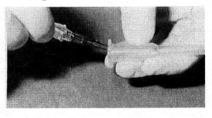

Angulation of the needle
using the catheter hub.

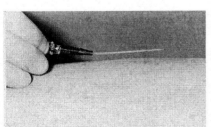

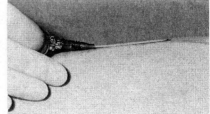

Forearm vein cannulation: Angulating the catheter prior to insertion
permits insertion of the cannula in the same plane as the vein.

Fig. 4: Note that vein immobilization is maintained throughout iv insertion.

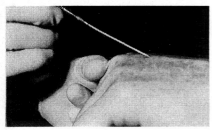
Puncture skin at 30 - 45°

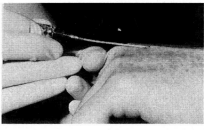
Decrease angle of insertion.

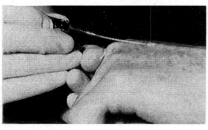
Blood flashes back into cannula hub as the vein is entered.

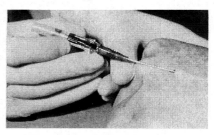
Advance another 2 - 3 mm to ensure catheter is in the vein.

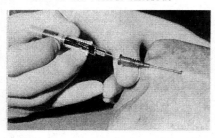
Catheter is left in the vein while the needle is withdrawn 1 cm.

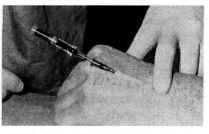
With the needle back 1 cm, the catheter is advanced to the hub.

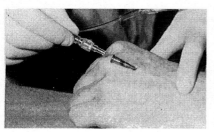

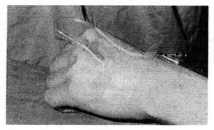

Once the vein is occluded (to prevent back-bleeding), the needle is removed and the iv tubing is connected. The iv is then secured with tape.

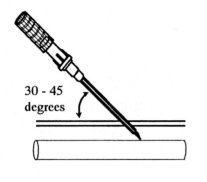

30 - 45
degrees

Puncture the skin holding the needle at a 30 - 45 degree angle and advance the needle until the catheter tip is beneath the skin.

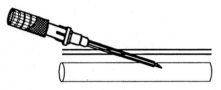

Decrease the angle of the intravenous catheter in relation to the vein. Watch for blood in the iv hub as the vein is entered.

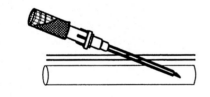

Advance the needle and catheter another 2 mm to ensure the catheter is in the vein.

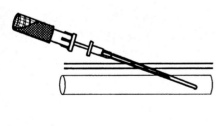

Without moving the catheter, withdraw the needle approximately 1 cm back from the tip of the catheter. Now advance both the catheter and needle into the vein.

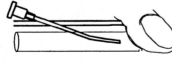

Release the tourniquet. Occlude the vein proximal to the catheter tip. Remove the needle, and secure the intravenous tubing to the catheter.

Figure 5: Establishing peripheral intravenous access.

Problems with Intravenous cannulation:

1. *Resistance is felt when attempts are made to advance the catheter over the needle.*

The most likely problem is the catheter is outside or only partially through the wall of the vein. Make sure that the needle and catheter are advanced approximately 2 mm into the vein after the flash back occurs so that the catheter will be in the vein before attempts are made to advance the catheter over the needle. If the catheter is at a sharp angle to the vein you will only have a short distance before the tip of the needle is through the vein when it is advanced. To avoid this, try to lower the angle of the catheter to keep it in the same plane as the vein.

2. *A large hematoma develops when attempting to insert the intravenous.*

A hematoma may develop whenever the vein is entered. This may occur when injecting local anaesthetic if the local is injected beneath the skin and into the vein. By injecting local anaesthetic immediately lateral to the vein, the chance of causing a hematoma is less. If a hematoma results while you are attempting to insert the intravenous, and your ability to visualize the vein is lost, you should remove the catheter and apply pressure with a gauze to prevent further bleeding. Release the tourniquet, and hold the site for a couple of minutes before trying again at another site.

3. *You advance the catheter easily into the vein but then encounter resistance before it is completely inserted.*

The catheter tip is likely lying next to a valve or junction in the vein. Do not force the catheter, you may be able to connect the catheter to the intravenous tubing and advance the catheter once fluid is flowing through the tubing. If not, you may still be able to achieve adequate administration of fluids and medications without having the catheter advanced all the way into the vein.

4. *The patient experiences excessive pain when inserting the intravenous.*

The intravenous needle and catheter may be dissecting along the vein wall. The vessel walls have sensory fibres and if the needle scrapes along the wall rather than entering it cleanly, the patient may experience significant pain with even a small intravenous. Other possibilities include nerve injury with needle insertion (e.g., median nerve in the anticubital fossa, radial nerve in the anatomical snuff box). Remove the intravenous and use an alternative site with local anaesthesia.

5. *Unable to enter the vein with the intravenous catheter.*

Inadequate stabilization of the vein is the most common mistake made when learning to insert an intravenous. Immobilize the vein by applying skin traction distal to the vein. Try to visualize where the tip of the needle is in relation to the vein. Lift the tip of the needle up so that you can see its relation to the vein. Line up the needle direction and plane with that of the vein. If you have advanced the needle and cannot enter the vein, withdraw the needle and catheter such that the catheter tip is just below the skin, and start again, adjusting to a different angle and depth. With time, the needle may become obstructed by clotted blood preventing a flash back from occuring when the needle is in the vein. Consider changing the intravenous needle and catheter after attempting catheterization for several minutes.

Other helpful hints:

To approximate the plane of the intravenous catheter with the plane of the vein being cannulated, it is often useful to create a slight (10 - 15 degree) angulation in the iv catheter before inserting it. This is particularly useful in cannulation of veins of the forearm, where it is difficult to hold the catheter at a low enough angle to approximate the plane of the iv catheter with the vein (figure 6).

The plastic iv housing unit which is supplied with the iv catheter can be used to create this angle just distal to the catheter hub. Angulate the catheter such that the bevel is facing up. The angulation allows the catheter hub to be held at a comfortable angle, and matches the plane of the iv catheter with the vein.

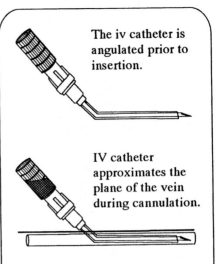

The iv catheter is angulated prior to insertion.

IV catheter approximates the plane of the vein during cannulation.

Figure 6:
Cannulation of forearm veins: Angulating the iv catheter prior to insertion may decrease the chance of passing through the back wall of the vein during cannulation.

Review Questions

Chapter 3:
Preoperative assessment.

1. Define the ASA physical status classification.
2. How long should elective surgery be postponed following a myocardial infarction? What is the basis of this recommendation?
3. What information should be obtained in the anaesthetic history?
4. What common anaesthetic techniques can be used to provide anaesthesia for lower abdominal surgery?
5. What anaesthetic risks might be associated in a patient who smokes regularly? What information obtained from history, physical, or laboratory examination might be useful in assessing this risk? Are there any means of decreasing the risks of perioperative complications related to smoking?

Chapter 4:
Premedication.

1. Why are patients premedicated prior to surgery?
2. What are the general contra-indications to the use of benzodiazepine or opioid pre-medications?

Chapter 6:
Intubation and anatomy of the airway.

1. What is the *"1-2-3"* test?
2. What does a class I hypopharyngeal view mean? What structures are visualized in a class I hypo-pharyngeal view?
3. What structures are visualized in a grade III laryngeal view?
4. What is the optimal position of the head and neck for intubation using direct laryngoscopy?
5. How is tracheal intubation confirmed?
6. Name 4 simple maneuvers that can be used to overcome an upper airway obstruction.

Chapter 7:
Intubation decisions.

1. What laboratory criteria should you use to assess the objective need for intubation and ventilation?
2. What are some important historical and clinical factors that suggest the need to intubate and ventilate a patient?

Chapter 8:
Laryngeal mask airway.

1. What is the difference between a LMA and an endotracheal tube?

2. Why would a laryngeal mask airway be used rather than a endotracheal tube?

Chapter 9:
Rapid sequence induction.

1. What is the purpose of a rapid
   sequence induction?
2. Describe the sequence of maneuvers
   used in a rapid sequence induction.
3. What is the purpose of pre-
   oxygenation?
4. Which patients should be regarded
   as being at risk of pulmonary aspiration of gastric contents?
5. What measures can be taken to
   decrease the risk of aspiration?

Chapter 10:
Monitoring in anaesthesia.

1. What information does the anaesthetist use to assess the depth of
   anaesthesia?
2. What information can be obtained
   by monitoring the capnograph?
3. What relationship does the ETCO2
   value have to the PaCO2? What
   conditions might result in a ETCO2
   measurement of 20 mm Hg with a
   PaCO2 measurement of 40 mm Hg?

Chapter 11:
Intravenous anaesthetic agents.

1. Why do patients awaken from a
   sleep dose of thiopental within 5 to
   10 minutes of its administration
   when the elimination half life is of
   the order of 5 - 12 hours?

2. Why would one choose propofol
   over thiopental as an intravenous
   induction agent?
3. When would one choose ketamine
   over either thiopental or propofol as
   the intravenous induction drug?
4. What are the concentrations and
   induction doses of thiopental and
   propofol?

Chapter 12:
Muscle relaxants.

1. What is the difference between a
   depolarizing and non-depolarizing
   muscle relaxant? Give examples of
   each.
2. What are the absolute contraindications to the use of succinylcholine?
3. Which patients are susceptible to
   hyperkalemia following succinylcholine?
4. What is the concentration that succinylcholine is supplied? What is the
   dose for intubation?
5. Which drugs can be used to
   antagonize a neuromuscular block?

Chapter 13:
Inhalational anaesthetic agents.

1. What is MAC?
2. What is the relationship between the
   anaesthetic concentration that is set
   on the anaesthetic vaporizer and the
   anaesthetic concentration in the
   patient's brain?
3. What is diffusion hypoxia?
4. What are the MAC values of isoflurane, enflurane, and halothane in
   oxygen?

Chapter 14:
Narcotic agonists and antagonists.

1. What undesirable effects do opioids have?
2. Name an opioid antagonist. What dose of this drug would be appropriate to reverse opioid induced respiratory depression. What, if any, are there any potential problems of giving too much of this antagonist?

Chapter 15:
Local and regional anaesthesia.

1. Name two classes of local anaesthetic agents, and give examples of each.
2. What is PABA, and what role does it have in local anaesthesia?
3. Name 4 techniques of administering a local anaesthetic drug.
4. Why is a vasoconstrictor often used with a local anaesthetic? Give an example of a LA vasoconstrictor and its concentration. When would the use of a vasoconstrictor be contraindicated?
5. Which regional block results in the highest concentration of local anaesthetic in the blood?
6 What is the maximum recommended dose of plain lidocaine, and of lidocaine with a vasoconstrictor?
7. Why might a regional anaesthetic be given as well as a general anaesthetic?
8. Describe some of the signs and symptoms of local anaesthetic toxicity.
9. Describe the steps in treating an acute local anaesthetic toxicity.

10. What is the difference between a spinal and an epidural anaesthetic?
11. How many milligrams of lidocaine are in 20 mls of a 2% solution?

Chapter 16:
Acute pain management.

1. List the physiological effects of acute pain.
2. Contrast intramuscular and PCA opioid administration.
3. What are the adverse effects resulting from the administration of excessive opioid analgesics?
4. What non-opioid analgesic agents are available for the control of acute pain?
5. What are the contraindications to administering a non-steroidal anti-inflammatory drug?
6. List an appropriate dose and schedule for two common NSAID's used to control of acute pain.

Chapter 17:
Chronic pain.

1. What is the difference between acute and chronic pain?
2. What is RSD? What conditions may lead to the development of RSD?
3. What modalities are commonly used to treat RSD?
4. How is a diagnosis of RSD made?
5. What are trigger points?
6. Name two surgical conditions that may present with back pain and require emergency surgical intervention ?

Chapter 18:
Obstetrical anaesthesia.

1. What is the supine hypotensive syndrome? How can it be prevented?
2. What factors may influence a patient's experience of pain during labour and delivery?
3. What options are available for dealing with the pain of labour and delivery?
4. What are the major risks of general anaesthesia in the parturient undergoing a cesarian section?

Chapter 19:
Basic neonatal resuscitation.

1. What is the Apgar score of a baby that is limp, blue, has no response to oropharyngeal suctioning, a heart rate of 60 bpm, and irregular gasping respiratory efforts?
2. Describe the basic steps in neonatal resuscitation.
3. When is positive pressure ventilation (PPV) indicated in the newborn infant? Describe the technique of PPV.
4. Assuming a newborn infant weighs 3 kg, what is the concentration and dose of epinephrine, and how ought it be administered?

Chapter 20:
Intravenous fluid and blood component therapy.

1. How are the hourly and daily maintenance fluid requirements calculated?

2. List conditions that may be associated with a significant preoperative fluid deficit.
3. What is the difference between a crystalloid and a colloid? Give examples of each.
4. Which patients should consider autologous blood donation? For which patients is this not suitable?
5. Calculate the acceptable amount of blood that can be lost in a 70 kg male if his initial hemoglobin is 140 gm/dl, and the accepted minimal hemoglobin after surgery is 80 gm/dl.
6. What is the most common cause of an ABO incompatible blood transfusion?
7. Name three different blood components that may be transfused.

Chapter 21:
Common perioperative problems.

1. Define shock? Classify the different types of shock and give examples of each.
2. What are some treatable causes of an agitated postoperative state?

Chapter 22:
Managing the circulation.

1. What are the broad goals in controlling the circulation?
2. What are the differences between an alpha-1 and beta-1 adrenergic agonist? Give examples of each.
3. What are the factors which determine cardiac output?

Chapter 23:
Oxygen therapy and hypoxia.

1. List some devices that are commonly used to deliver oxygen to spontaneously breathing patients.
2. When should a puritan face mask be used? When should one use a manual resuscitation device, such as an Ambu bag and mask unit?
3. List the five categories of conditions causing hypoxemia.
4. List the four categories of conditions causing hypoxia.

Chapter 24:
Unusual anaesthetic complications.

1. What is MH?
2. List two anaesthetic agents that may trigger an MH reaction.
3. Which drug is used specifically to treat an MH reaction?
4. What strategies are useful in reducing the perioperative risk of pulmonary aspiration of gastric contents?
5. Describe the steps used to treat an anaphylactic reaction.

Index

Notes